Blood Groups:
P, I, Sd^a and Pr

Mention of specific products or equipment by contributors to this American Association of Blood Banks publication does not represent an endorsement of such products by the American Association of Blood Banks, nor does it necessarily indicate a preference for those products over other similar competitive products.

Efforts are made to have publications of the AABB consistent in regard to acceptable practices. However, for several reasons, they may not be. First, as new developments in the practice of blood banking occur, changes may be recommended to the *Standards for Blood Banks and Transfusion Services*. It is not possible, however, to revise each publication at the time such a change is adopted. Thus, it is essential that the most recent edition of the *Standards* be used as the ultimate reference in regard to current acceptable practices. Second, the views expressed in this publication represent the opinions of the authors and do not reflect the official policy of the American Association of Blood Banks or the institution with which the author is affiliated, unless this is clearly specified.

Blood Groups:
P, I, Sd^a and Pr

Editors

Joann M. Moulds, PhD
Research Fellow
Washington University School of Medicine
St. Louis, Missouri

Laura Lee Woods, MS, MT(ASCP)SBB
Supervisor, Blood Bank
Baptist Memorial Hospital
Memphis, Tennessee

American Association of Blood Banks
Arlington, Virginia
1991

Copyright © 1991 by the American Association of Blood Banks. All rights reserved. No part of this book may be reproduced or transmitted in any form or by any means, electronic or mechanical, including photocopying, recording, or by any information storage and retrieval system, without permission in writing from the Publisher.

American Association of Blood Banks
1117 North 19th Street, Suite 600
Arlington, Virginia 22209

ISBN NO. 1-56395-002-2
Printed in the United States

Library of Congress Cataloging-in-Publication Data

Blood groups: P, I, Sd^a and Pr/Editors,
JoAnn M. Moulds, Laura Lee Woods
p. cm.
Includes bibliographical references and index.
ISBN 1-56395-002-2 (hardcover)
1. Blood groups—Analysis. 2. Compatibility testing (Hematology).
I. Moulds, Jo Ann. II. Woods, Laura Lee.
[DNLM: 1. Antigens. 2. Blood Grouping and Crossmatching.
3. Blood Groups. WH 420 B6558]
RB45.5.B56 1991
612.1'1825—dc20
DNLM/DLC
for Library of Congress

91-4870
CIP

Technical/Scientific Workshops Committee

Dennis M. Smith, Jr., MD, Chairman

Michael L. Baldwin, MBA, MT(ASCP)SBB
Alice Reynolds Barr, SBB(ASCP)
Daniel B. Brubaker, DO
Katherine B. Carlson, MT(ASCP)SBB
Morris R. Dixon, MS, MT(ASCP)SBB
Frances L. Gibbs, MS, MT(ASCP)SBB
Christina A. Kasprisin, MS, RN
Sanford R. Kurtz, MD
Barbara Laird-Fryer, MT(ASCP)SBB
Judith S. Levitt, MT(ASCP)SBB
Leo J. McCarthy, MD
JoAnn M. Moulds, PhD
Ronald A. Sacher, MD
Phyllis Unger, MT(ASCP)SBB
Robert G. Westphal, MD
Susan M. Wilson, MT(ASCP)SBB
Laura Lee Woods, MS, MT(ASCP)SBB

Contents

Foreword ix

1. **The P Blood Group System: Biochemistry, Genetics and Clinical Significance** 1

   Harold B. Anstall, MD, and Robert C. Blaylock, MD

   Biochemistry and Genetics of the P Blood Group System 2
   Antibodies Directed Against P System Antigenic Determinants 12
   The Clinical Significance of the P Blood Group System and Its Antibodies 15
   Conclusion 19
   References 19

2. **The I Blood Group Collection** 23

   Malcolm L. Beck, FIMLS, MIBiol

   Serologic History 24
   Genetics and Biochemistry 32
   Pathologic Significance 35
   Summary 45
   References 45

3. **The Antigens Sd^a and Cad** 53

   Peter D. Issitt, PhD, FIMLS, FIBiol, CBiol, FRCPath

   Sd^a 54
   Cad 60
   Biochemistry 61
   References 68

4. **Cold-Reactive Autoantibodies Outside the I and P Blood Groups** 73

   Peter D. Issitt, PhD, FIMLS, FIBiol, CBiol, FRCPath

   The Pr Antigens 73
   Antigens Defined by Other Cold Agglutinins 88
   A Brief Summary of the Antigens Pr, Gd, Sa, Fl, Lud, Vo, Li, IgM^{woo}, Me, Om and Ju 95
   The Antigen Rx 98
   Unnamed Antigens Defined by Cold Agglutinins 101
   References 101

5. **Serology of P, I, Sd^a, Rx and Pr** 113
   Marilyn K. Moulds, MT(ASCP)SBB

   P 113
   I 117
   Sd^a 122
   Pr 125
   Summary 127
   References 128
   Appendix 5-1. Donath-Landsteiner Test 133
   Appendix 5-2. Inhibition of Anti-P1 135
   Appendix 5-3. Inhibition of Anti-I 137
   Appendix 5-4. Cold Autoantibody Absorption With
      Formaldehyde-Fixed Rabbit Red Blood Cells or Rabbit
      Stroma 139
   Appendix 5-5. Inhibition of Anti-Sd^a 141
   Appendix 5-6. Preparation of Ficin and Trypsin 143
   Appendix 5-7. Preparation of Löw's Cysteine-Activated Papain .. 144
   Appendix 5-8. Standardization of Enzyme Solutions for
      Two-Stage Technique 145
   Appendix 5-9. Neuraminidase Treatment of Red Cells 147

Index 149

Foreword

This book represents the continuation of the series on blood group systems. However, the astute reader will note that not all the blood groups covered in this publication are systems as recently defined by the International Society of Blood Transfusion (ISBT) Working Party on Terminology for Red Cell Surface Antigens. Rather, the groups contained herein have been brought together in this book because their antibodies characteristically react at room temperature or below—ie, cold agglutinins.

In order to be consistent with established policies, the authors have attempted to use the ISBT nomenclature when appropriate. However, this is particularly difficult for the P blood group system as several antigens, historically linked to P1, have not been convincingly proven to be genetically related and thus have not been assigned system numbers. Therefore, the reader will find a mixture of "old" and "new" terminology in this book.

The expert serologists who have authored these chapters do an outstanding job in reviewing the historical aspects of the P blood group system and the Ii blood group collection, as well as Sd^a, Rx, Pr and other miscellaneous cold agglutinins. The reasons for renaming and reassigning antigens and antibodies are discussed in relation to currently known biochemical facts. Although many transfusion services no longer perform room temperature antibody screens or compatibility tests, cold agglutinins may still present problems as they go unrecognized. The chapter on serologic techniques discusses some of these problems and presents methods for dealing with cold-reactive antibodies.

The information provided in this book should be useful for both the entry-level technologist as well as those wishing a more in-depth knowledge of these blood groups.

JoAnn M. Moulds, PhD
Laura Lee Woods, MS, MT(ASCP)SBB
Editors

In: Moulds JM and Woods LL, eds.
Blood Groups: P, I, Sd^a and Pr
Arlington, VA: American Association of Blood Banks, 1991

1

The P Blood Group System: Biochemistry, Genetics and Clinical Significance

Harold B. Anstall, MD, and
Robert C. Blaylock, MD

THE P BLOOD GROUP SYSTEM was discovered by Landsteiner and Levine in 1927 during the course of animal experiments in which rabbits were variously inoculated with red cells derived from several humans. Rabbit serum was subsequently harvested and screened against human red cells for antihuman antibody formation. One positive result of these experiments was the production of an antibody defining a hitherto unrecognized antigen now called P1, designated by the code number 003001 in the numerical nomenclature recently adopted by the International Society for Blood Transfusion.[1-7] This nomenclature represents a truly significant effort to classify group antigens in a logical and systematic manner, taking biochemical, genetic and immunologic characteristics into full consideration. This has led to the reorientation and reassignment of some antigens, and to the renaming of some former blood group systems. In this context, the P blood group system is now designated P1 (003). The definitive antigen of this system (defined by the antibody anti-P1) is identified, therefore, by the numerical symbol 003001.[6]

Other antigenic entities defined by specific antibodies found in human sera have been described and include P, P^k and p. P, P^k and Luke have been assigned to the globoside collection of antigens (209) and given the ISBT numbers 209001, 209002 and 209003, respectively (JJ Moulds, Chairman, ISBT Working Party on Terminology, personal communication). At the date of writing, p has not been assigned a definitive code number in the ISBT nomenclature.[6] The relationship to the P1 (003) system—genetically

---

Harold B. Anstall, MD, Professor of Pathology and Robert C. Blaylock, MD, Fellow in Transfusion Medicine, Department of Pathology, University of Utah College of Medicine, Salt Lake City, Utah

and biochemically—will be addressed in subsequent sections of this chapter.

Biochemistry and Genetics of the P Blood Group System

Characteristically, antigenic specificities in the P system are determined by well-defined oligosaccharide sequences, primarily linked to the linear fatty acid chain of sphingolipids of the cell membrane. The sequence and steric attachment of the constituent carbohydrate molecules in these oligosaccharide chains define the haptenic specificities of the respective antigens. These definitive steric attachments are brought about by gene-specified glycosyltransferases, which are themselves the products of structural genes encoding for the various antigenic determinants associated with the system.

Distribution of P1 Antigens in Nature

The relatively widespread distribution of P system antigens in other biological species (particularly the P1 antigen itself) led to considerable interest in these glycolipids, which resulted in a substantial investigative effort.[8] This in turn led to considerable understanding of the biochemical structure of the P system antigens in general and of P1 in particular. It had been known for many years that P1-specific substance could be found in hydatid cyst fluid in patients with hydatid disease (*Echinococcus granulosus*), and that many such patients developed in their plasma an antibody with strong anti-P1 activity.[4,9] The fairly frequent presence of a similar antibody in patients harboring the liver fluke *Fasciola hepatica* and related species suggests the presence of the corresponding antigen (P1) among at least some species of trematodes.[4] In all cases where anti-P1 antibody was found in these various patients, their red cells were of the P_2 phenotype; ie, they were negative for the P1 antigen.

The P1 antigen has been isolated from other sources including mammalian tissues, pigeons and related species of birds and certain bacteria.[4,10,11] In the human body, P system antigens are found abundantly on red cells, granulocytes, lymphocytes and platelets.[4] They are also found on a variety of other cells, and in particular on uroepithelium, where the presence of P1 and P^k receptors plays a significant role in the pathogenesis of certain cases of pyelonephritis.[11] This widespread distribution of P system antigens among widely diverse species is a good example of the often-observed ubiquity of certain kinds of molecular species—in this case, glycosphingolipids.

Structure of P1 System Antigens

The P1 antigenic determinant and the other determinants formerly associated with the P blood group system are glycosphingolipids. The biochemical origin and structure of glycosphingolipids are illustrated in Fig 1-1. They are derivatives of ceramide, which is built up from the base sphingosine and a long-chain fatty acid of variable length. Monosaccharide units may then be added to the free hydroxyl group of the sphingosine moiety. In the context of "P system" specificities, the basic precursor is ceramide dihexoside (lactosylceramide), consisting of ceramide linked through the sphingosine oxygen function to glucose, which in turn is linked to galactose through a $\beta(1 \rightarrow 4)$ linkage. Thus, in common with the antigenic determinants of the ABO (001), H (018) and Le (007) systems, the antigens found on red cells are carried on Type II chains, specified by the $\beta(1 \rightarrow 4)$ linkage between the glucose and galactose of ceramide dihexoside (Type 2 chain).[4,11,12]

From this basic precursor structure two short series of antigens are synthesized by the appropriate action of gene-specified glycosyl-transferases—the globoside series (P^k, P and the Forssman antigen) and the paragloboside series comprising the P1 antigen and the p-specific determinant. The structures of these various antigenic species are illustrated graphically in Fig 1-2 and Fig 1-3. Figure 1-2 shows the globoside series. Beginning with ceramide dihexoside (CDH) as the precursor, a P^k or P^{1k}-gene-specified glycosyltransferase adds a second galactose in an $\alpha(1 \rightarrow 4)$ position to the two monosaccharide units already present, forming ceramide trihexoside (CTH), or P^k antigen. Through this the further addition of a molecule of N-acetylgalactosamine in a $\beta(1 \rightarrow 3)$ position forms globoside, which is identical to P. The addition of N-acetylgalactose to the terminal sugar of globoside in the $\alpha(2 \rightarrow 3)$ position gives rise to the Forssman structure.

Figure 1-3 shows the paragloboside series. Paragloboside is the precursor for the definitive antigen of the P blood group system—P1—and of the structure to which p specificity is assigned. It is formed by the addition of a galactose to the terminal N-acetylglucosamine in the $\beta(1 \rightarrow 4)$ position. To this structure, a P^{1k}-specified transferase adds a terminal galactose in the $\alpha(1 \rightarrow 4)$ position, forming the P1 antigen. The same enzyme converts CDH to P^k. Paragloboside may be modified in another direction, namely by adding N-acetylneuraminic acid to the terminal galactose in an $\alpha(2 \rightarrow 3)$ position. This addition gives rise to the p specificity, or sialosylparagloboside. It is felt that the gene specifying the transferase that brings about this final edition of N-acetylneuraminic acid is independent of the P system.

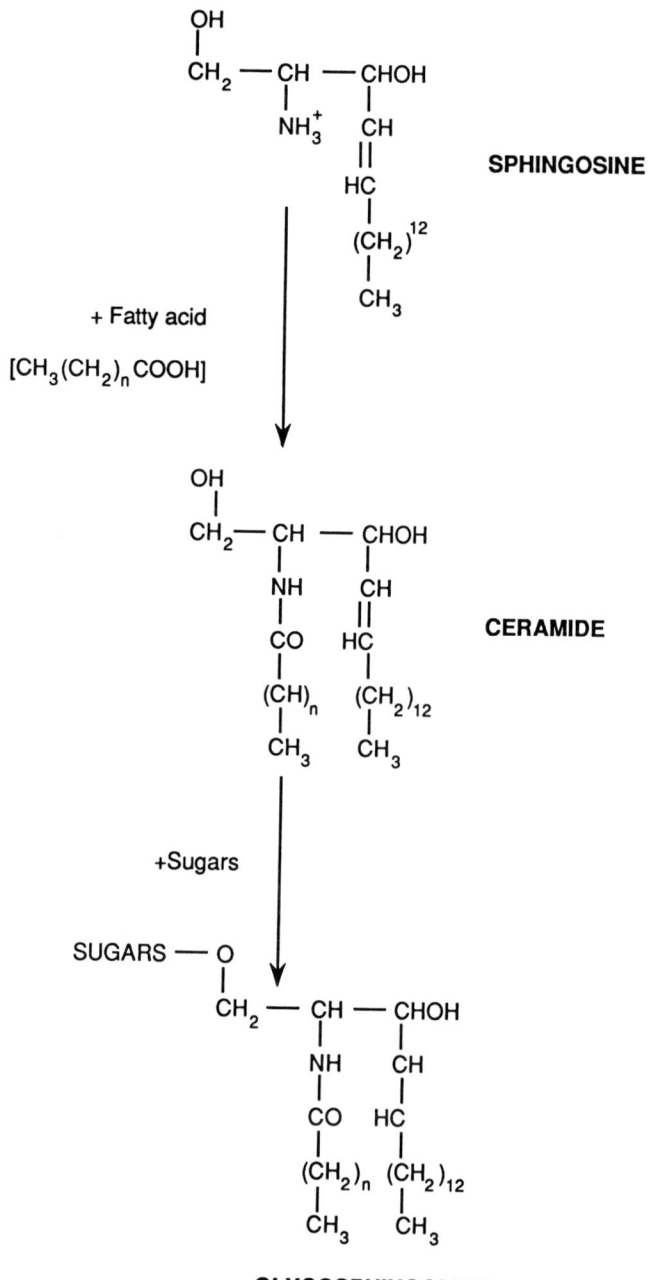

Figure 1-1. The origin and basic structure of glycolipid antigens.

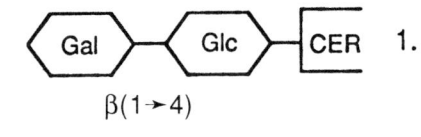

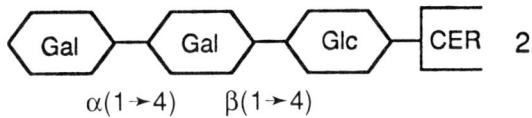

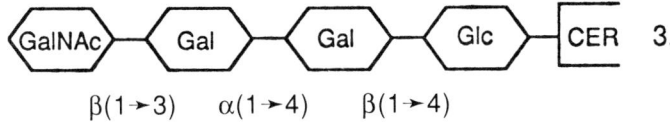

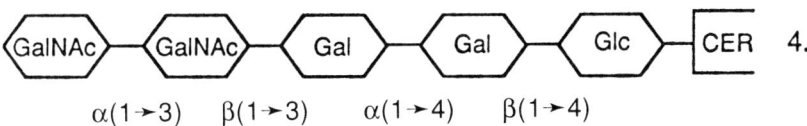

1. Ceramide Dihexoside (Lactosylceramide)

2. Ceramide Trihexoside (P^k)

3. Globoside (P)

4. Forssman Structures

Figure 1-2. Ceramide precursors, globoside and the Forssman structure.

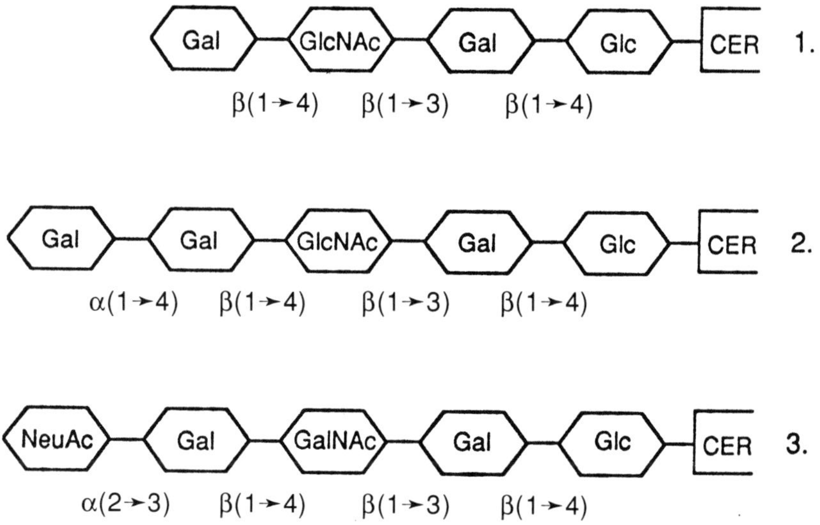

6 BLOOD GROUPS: P, I, Sd^a AND Pr

Gal —β(1→4)— GlcNAc —β(1→3)— Gal —β(1→4)— Glc — CER   1.

Gal —α(1→4)— Gal —β(1→4)— GlcNAc —β(1→3)— Gal —β(1→4)— Glc — CER   2.

NeuAc —α(2→3)— Gal —β(1→4)— GalNAc —β(1→3)— Gal —β(1→4)— Glc — CER   3.

1. Paragloboside

2. P1 Antigen

3. p Determinant (Sialosylparagloboside)

Figure 1-3. Paragloboside and the P1 (003001) and p determinants.

P System Genetics and the Formation of Antigenic Specificities

The formation of the various antigenic specificities from CDH and CTH precursors seems to fit the biochemical facts closely. However, some apparent anomalies both in the serologic behavior of some antibodies detected in the sera of people lacking certain of these antigens, together with other biochemical curiosities apparently observed on red cells themselves, have made these ostensibly simple synthetic models somewhat difficult to reconcile with a clear-cut model of gene action.

For example, if we consider the two most common phenotypes of the P system, which together account for 99.9% of the population between them and the P specificity on their red cells, it will be seen that all the biochemical evidence points to the synthesis of P from P^k (CTH). However, it is generally not possible to demonstrate presence of the P^k specificity on the red cells of these phenotypes (P_1 and P_2). Usually, when one antigen is converted to another on the red cell membrane, it is possible to demonstrate small residual amounts of the immediate precursor remaining after the greater part has been transformed into the new antigenic species.

Failure to do this in the case of the $P^k \rightarrow P$ conversion led to some difficulty in reconciling this transformation with a comprehensive genetic model.

On the other hand, although persons of the P_1 and P_2 phenotype apparently do not possess P^k, no persons of either phenotype appear capable of forming an anti-P^k antibody.[13] Indeed, anti-P^k activity is found only in persons of the p phenotype who form either anti-P + P_1 or anti-P + P_1 + P^k! Again, the frequency of the so-called P^k gene in the population appears to be exceedingly rare, so that the P_1k phenotype is very seldom seen.

Thus, it is difficult to explain the fact that the overwhelming majority of persons have P-positive red cells if the formation of P is dependent upon a glycosyltransferase that is specified by a gene of apparently great rarity.[13,14] Family studies also suggest that in the inheritance of the P system antigens, two loci appear to be involved. The P^1, P^2 and P genes appeared to behave as alleles at one such locus, but p seemed associated with another.[4,13,14] A further mystery is seen in the case of some persons whose red cells are positive for the P^k antigen (CTH). Some of these people are positive for P^k and P1 specificities (P_1k phenotype) and others for P^k alone (P_2k phenotype). In neither case, however, is P specificity demonstrable on their red cells! While conversion of P^k to P could be explained by postulating the absence of a specific P-gene-determined transferase in these persons, the occurrence of P1-positive and P1-negative red cells respectively in the presence of P^k antigen (CTH) suggested that P^1 and P^k genes were expressed at different loci.

Whereas several hypotheses have been advanced to explain these and other apparent serologic anomalies with respect to the P system,[13-15] the model proposed by Graham and Williams provides a most plausible means for reconciling the observed biochemical data with a workable genetic schema. This is illustrated in simplified form in Fig 1-4.[4,15]

The model is based upon the sequential action of gene products specified by genes at two loci, indicated as first locus and second locus in the illustration. The sequential action of gene-specified glycosyltransferases derived respectively from first and second locus genes upon two basic precursor substances—CDH and paragloboside—is considered. Genes considered to be situated at the first locus include P^{1k}, P^k and p. Those considered to be situated at the second locus include P^2 and $P^{2.0}$. The eventual antigenic specificities that appear on the red cell membrane glycosphingolipids depend upon what modification (if any) of the structures resulting from the action of the first locus genes (if any) is brought about by the enzymic products of the second locus genes. The following sequences are illustrated:

1. The action of the enzymic product of the P^{1k} gene on CDH is to convert it to CTH by the addition of a terminal D-galactose in an $\alpha(1 \rightarrow 4)$ position. It will be recalled that this structure is also known as the P^k antigen. If this structure now encounters the enzymic product of the second locus gene P^2, it is converted virtually completely to the P antigenic determinant by the

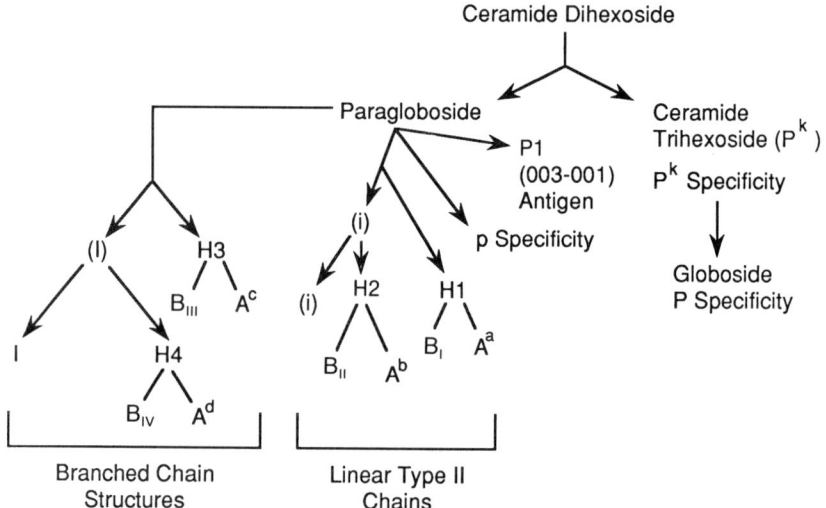

Figure 1-4. Interrelationships between the pathways of formation of the antigenic determinants of the P1 (003), H (018) and ABO (001) blood group systems.

addition of a terminal N-acetyl-D-galactosamine in the $\beta(1\to3)$ position to the P^k structure. If, instead of a P^2 gene at the second locus, there is a $P^{2.0}$ gene (which is a postulated amorph), no conversion of the P^k determinant into P determinant will occur. Further, if the actions of the same enzymic gene product upon the substrate paragloboside are considered, the action of the first locus gene P^{1k} will be to convert directly into P1 antigen.

The enzymic product of the second locus gene P^2 has no effect on this substance, and P1 antigen will appear on the red cells. If no P^2 gene is present at the second locus, but only $P^{2.0}$, no modification of the P1 antigen will occur. From this description and a perusal of Table 1-1, it should be apparent that these sequences described will result in red cells of the P_1 and P_1k phenotypes, respectively. Thus, the red cells of the P_1 phenotype person carries the P_1 and P specificities, while the P_1k person carries P_1 and P^k on his/her red cells.

2. Where only a P^k gene is found at the first locus, CDH is converted virtually completely to P^k. Since the enzymic product of the second locus gene P^2 has no effect upon P^k, no further modification of this substance occurs. Also, since the P^k gene product has no effect upon paragloboside, no conversion to P1 antigen takes place. Therefore, the red cells of such rare persons carry only P^k determinant and are phenotypically called P_2k.

3. Persons homozygous for the p gene, proposed as a silent allele at the first locus, have red cells that test negatively for P1, P^k and P determinants. In other words, p persons lack $\alpha(1\to4)$ galactosyltransferase. However, such cells generally show a relative abundance of the designated p determinant, which appears to be synthesized from paragloboside by the addition of a terminal N-acetylneuraminic acid in an $\alpha(2\to3)$ position.[15] It does not

Table 1-1. A Postulated Series of Genetic Sequences to Explain the Expression of P1 (003) System Antigens on Red Cells Expressed Between Various Phenotypes

Precursor	First Locus Gene	Intermediate	Second Locus Gene	Converts	Specificities on RBC	Phenotype
Ceramide Dihexoside (CDH)	P^{1k}	CTH (P^k)	P^2	$P^k \to P$	P1P	P_1
Paragloboside	P^{1k}	P1	P^2	no effect		
CDH	P^{1k}	CTH (P^k)	$P^{2.0}$	no effect	P1P^k	P_1^k
Paragloboside	P^{1k}	P1	$P^{2.0}$	no effect		
CDH	P^k	CTH (P^k)	P^2	$P^k \to P$	P	P_2
Paragloboside	P^k	—	P^2	no effect		
CDH	P^k	CTH (P^k)	$P^{2.0}$	no effect	P^k	P_2^k
Paragloboside	P^k	—	$P^{2.0}$	no effect		
CDH	p	—	P^2 or $P^{2.0}$	no effect	—	p
Paragloboside	p	—	P^2 or $P^{2.0}$	no effect	p*	

*p is believed to be an amorph. p determinant is probably present in small amounts on all RBCs and in larger amounts in people of the p phenotype

appear that the so-called *p* gene codes for the specific transferase that brings about the formation of this determinant. Indeed, small amounts of this material (p) appear to be formed on most red cells regardless of the P system phenotype.[16]

It is more likely that the p determinant (sialosylparagloboside) is formed by the action of sialosyltransferases encoded by other structural genes unrelated to the P blood group system. Relatively large amounts of sialosylparagloboside are found on the red cells of p phenotype persons, probably because no other P system gene-specified enzymes are present to convert paragloboside into the various P system determinants. The relatively random action of sialosyltransferases encoded by unrelated genes is enhanced by the fact that an abundance of unconverted paragloboside is available to them as substrate, and larger amounts of sialosylparagloboside can be easily formed. If red cells of various P system phenotypes are tested with the few available examples of anti-p, cells of the p phenotype react strongly, whereas P_2 cells react more weakly and P_1 cells most weakly of all. This reflects the decreasing presence of the sialosylparagloboside on cells that possess gene-specified transferases capable of converting paragloboside into other entities.[17,18] In this context, therefore, so-called p determinant occurs fortuitously and should not really be considered a part of the P system.

It has been observed that the red cells of persons having the P^{1k} gene at the first locus generally exhibit more P^k determinant than do the red cells of persons who lack that gene at the first locus but who convert P^k to P because of the inheritance of a P^2 gene at the second locus. This may refer to differences in kinetic properties between the galactosyltransferases specified by the P^{1k} and P^k genes, respectively. The enzyme specified by the P^{1k} gene catalyzes the addition of D-galactose CDH $\alpha(1\rightarrow 4)$ position, thus converting it to P^k antigen; it adds the same monosaccharide in the same steric position to paragloboside, converting it to P1 antigen. The galactosyltransferase-specified first locus gene P^k differs from the above in that while it readily brings about the conversion of CDH through P^k antigen, it is unable to add a terminal D-galactose to paragloboside, and thus does not convert it to P1 antigen.[18,19] Whereas these differences presuppose differences in binding ability of the two transferases with respect to the different substrates involved in these conversions, there is also an implication that where the P^2 gene is present, the N-acetyl-D-galactosaminyltransferase that is coded for by the P^2 gene brings about a less complete conversion of P^k to globoside (P).

The distribution of P system phenotypes among the Black and White populations is illustrated in Table 1-2. A summary of P system genotypes according to the most plausible genetic model described above is shown in Table 1-3. This table serves to summarize the genotypic expression of antigens within this system with the conventional phenotypes, and to indicate in each case the expression of antigens on corresponding red cells.

Table 1-2. The Phenotypes of the P1 (003) Blood Group Systems

1st Locus Genotypes	2nd Locus Genotypes	Phenotype	Antigens on RBCs
$P^{1k}\ P^{1k}$ $P^{1k}\ P^k$ $P^{1k}\ P$	$P^2\ P^2$ or $P^2\ P^{2.0}$	P_1	P1, P
$P^{1k}\ P^{1k}$ $P^{1k}\ P^k$ $P^{1k}\ P$	$P^{2.0}P^{2.0}$	P_1^k	P1, P^k
$P^k\ P^k$ or $P^k p$	$P^2\ P^2$ $P^2\ P^{2.0}$	P_2	P
$P^k\ P^k$ or $P^k p$	$P^{2.0}\ P^{2.0}$	P_2^k	P^k
pp	any combination	p	sialosyl-paragloboside

The Luke (LKE) Antigen and Antibody

An unusual antibody, characterized anti-Luke, was described by Tippett et al in 1965. This hitherto undescribed antibody appeared to divide red cells into three phenotypic categories: Luke−, Luke (w) and Luke +. Because of the observation that all p and P^k red cells reacted negatively with anti-Luke antibody, there was an association between the Luke antigen (209003) and the P blood group system. However, examples of red cells were found that were not of the p or P^k phenotypes but were Luke−; also, the Luke− and Luke (w) phenotypes were more frequent among P1-negative than among P1-positive samples. Yet again, the Luke− and Luke (w) phenotypes were

Table 1-3. Relationship Between Genotypes Determined by First and Second Locus Genes, Phenotypes and Antigens Finally Expressed on RBCs

Cell Phenotype	React Positively with Anti-	Antigens on RBCs	Frequency % Whites	Frequency % Blacks
P_1	-P1, -P	P1, P	80	93
P_2	-P	P	20	7
P_1^k	-P1, $-P^k$	P1, P^k	v. rare	
P_2^k	$-P^k$	P^k	v. rare	
p	"anti-p"	Sialosylpara-globoside	v. rare	

more commonly found among A_1 than among A_2, B or O persons. It thus seems that the antigens of the ABO (001) system that are carried on the same membrane glycosphingolipid structures as the P system determinants affect the expression on red cells of the determinant defined by the anti-Luke antibody.[20] It is believed that the gene responsible for the expression of the Luke antigen segregates separately from genes of the P blood group system, and is therefore independent of that system.[20]

The *In(Lu)* Gene and Expression of the P1 Antigen

It has been known for some years that the gene *In(Lu)*—whose presence is suppressive to the expression of Lu^a and Lu^b antigens, but that is not located at the Lu locus—may also affect the expression of the P1 antigen.[20,21] Therefore, it seems that people who inherit the *In(Lu)* gene and the P^{1k} gene may well have red cells that are deficient in the expression of the P1 antigen, even though the P^{1k} gene and the *In(Lu)* genes are situated at totally different loci.

Antibodies Directed Against P System Antigenic Determinants

Since the serologic identification of the P system is discussed in detail in Chapter 5, this section gives a brief and general survey of the most significant characteristics of antibodies directed against P system antigens that are likely to be encountered in clinical practice, and may have some special clinical significance. The general properties of such antibodies are summarized briefly in Table 1-4. From Table 1-4, it will be apparent that certain features are generically characteristic of the antibodies with activity against determinants of this system: They are predominantly IgM in nature and, therefore, tend to be reactive in saline but not in protein media or by the antiglobulin reaction. Few cause in vitro hemolysis and the thermal optimum of many antibodies is significantly lower than ambient body temperature. On the other hand, there are exceptions to some of these features. A brief review of the principal antibodies encountered clinically in relation to the P system follows.

Anti-P1

This antibody is frequently encountered in the plasma of persons of the P_2 phenotype who lack the P1 antigen on their red cells. In keeping with the most usual characteristics of P system antibodies, most examples are IgM agglutinins that bring about relatively weak agglutination of P1-positive red cells at temperatures below 25 C in isotonic saline. Only occasional examples show IgG specificity, reacting in the antiglobulin test.[4] If the

Table 1-4. Characteristics of P1 (003) Blood Group System Antibodies

Antibody	Usual Mode of Reaction			Immunoglobulin Class		TRs		% Caucasians Positive
	Sal.	DAT*	IgM	IgG	Yes		HDN	
Anti-P1	+	Few	+	Few	Few		No	80
Anti-P^k	+		+		No		No	<1
Anti-P†	+		Most	Few	Yes			100
Anti-Tj^a (−P + P_1 + P^k)	+	Few	Most	Few	Yes		Yes	100
Anti-IP_1	+		+		No		No	80

*DAT—Direct Antiglobulin Test
†—includes Donath-Landsteiner Antibody

temperature of the test system is lowered further and the incubation time suitably prolonged, anti-P1 is discovered with increasing frequency in the sera of P_2 people—ultimately reaching more than 60%! It should be emphasized that the high incidence of this antibody in individuals of P_2 phenotype refers to weakly reacting, low-titer examples of the antibody in healthy persons generally with no transfusion history.

Much stronger examples of anti-P1 are found in people exposed to P1 or P1-like specific substances either by transfusion, through exposure to known sources of antigen or in certain diseases. Thus, antibody of higher titer and greater avidity, and sometimes of broader thermal range, can be found in persons of the P_2 phenotype with hydatid disease, and fascioliasis (bovine liver fluke) infestation. Virtually all show positivity for the presence of a potent anti-P1 in the sera, reflecting the presence of the corresponding antigen in hydatid cyst fluid and on the surface of the parasites. Again, the occurrence of this same antibody in the plasma of pigeon-breeders and handlers reflects the fact that these birds possess the corresponding antigen on their red cells, in their tissues and in their bodily secretions and droppings.

The clinical significance of anti-P1 in transfusion practice will be discussed later. Here it may simply be said that the antibody is rarely of much significance, is rarely implicated in transfusion reactions and is not associated with hemolytic disease of the newborn (HDN).

Anti-P

Virtually all cases of anti-P are found in sera of people of the P_1k and P_2k phenotypes, both of which lack the P determinant (globoside). The antibody reacts with all cells of the P_1 and P_2 phenotypes, but not with P^k or p red cells. As with anti-P1, such apparent isoantibodies are generally of low titer and avidity, and of low thermal amplitude. Anti-P1 may, however, appear as an alloantibody (eg, after transfusion with P-positive red cells) in persons of the P_1k or P_2k phenotypes, in which case it may be much more potent and may require such persons needing transfusion to receive only P-negative red cells.[4]

The autoantibody with anti-P activity originally described by Donath and Landsteiner and associated with paroxysmal cold hemoglobinuria (PCH) will be discussed later in this chapter.

Anti-Tj^a (Anti-P + P_1 + P^k)

This antibody occurs spontaneously in persons of the p phenotype. It was originally considered to be an antibody directed against an antigen of very high incidence, originally called Tj^a,[4] now known to be capable of interacting with the P antigens P, P1 and P^k. As we have already seen, the p phenotype is very rare, with perhaps a slightly higher frequency of occurrence among Japanese populations.[4]

The antibody—uniformly present in the plasma of persons of p phenotype—appears to be a mixture of anti-P, anti-P1 and anti-P^k. The antibody is absent at birth in newborns of the p phenotype, but develops in similar fashion to the anti-A and anti-B isoagglutinins over several months following delivery. Although a majority of examples are IgM in character, some are IgG. Antibody may act as a potent in vitro hemolysin, and has been associated with severe hemolytic transfusion reactions.[22] Because some examples of this antibody are IgG in character, it has been reported as a cause of HDN. Further aspects of the clinical significance of this antibody are discussed later in this chapter.

Anti-p

Several workers have reported examples of antibodies that, while reacting weakly with cells of the P_1 and P_2 phenotypes and occurring transiently in the sera of persons of the P_1 phenotype, react preferentially with cells of the p phenotype. These antibodies generally develop in the convalescent stage of a respiratory illness, and survive in the serum for only a limited time. They appear to interact with the p-specific substance that appears to be formed by a glycosyltransferase coded for by a gene independent of the P blood group system. While being present to some extent on virtually all red cells, this p-specific substance is most abundant on cells of the p phenotype, for reasons discussed previously.[22] It is assumed that the antibody is formed in response to an antigen borne by a viral agent similar to or identical with the p determinant and cross-reacting with it.

Other Polyclonal Antibodies

Antibodies with anti-IP_1, anti-iP_1, anti-I^TP_1 and anti-iP specificities have been described.[23-26] The occurrence of such specificity serves further to indicate that the antigenic determinants of ABO (001), H (018), Ii (207) and P1 are closely interrelated and borne upon the same basic glycosphingolipid membrane-associated structures.

The Clinical Significance of the P Blood Group System and Its Antibodies

The Clinical Significance of Anti-P1 in Transfusion Practice

It has become clear from experience widely reported in the literature[27,28] that most examples of anti-P1 are of minor, if any, clinical significance. It seems that those antibodies not reactive at 37 C, and certainly those with temperature optima less than 30 C do not significantly shorten the life span of P1-positive red cells.[20,25] Concerns that the transfusion of P1-positive red cells into persons whose plasma contains anti-P1 activity (even with a low thermal range) could stimulate an anamnestic increase in titer or a broadening of the thermal amplitude of the antibody appear to be without foundation.[29-32] Further, intravenous injection of small amounts of P1-positive red cells into persons with warm-reactive (optimum 37 C) antibody did not have any adverse result.[32] In general, it is probably true to say that regardless of the presence of anti-P1 activity in recipient serum, if compatibility testing at 37 C is nonreactive, then transfusion of the corresponding P1-positive donor red cells will not result in a transfusion reaction or in a measurable reduction in posttransfusion life span of the donor cells.

However, it should be pointed out that those examples of anti-P1 that can be shown to fix complement at 37 C, and are likewise crossmatch-incompatible in the antiglobulin reaction at that temperature, should be considered clinically significant and potentially dangerous.

Anti-P + P_1 + P^k and Malignant Disease

The original description of anti-P + P_1 + P^k in a patient of the p phenotype was that of a woman suffering from gastric carcinoma.[4] This condition is generally associated with a very high mortality and a negligible 5-year survival rate. However, in this particular case, removal of the tumor by partial gastrectomy resulted in complete recovery, the patient surviving into late old age and dying of unrelated causes more than two decades after the surgery. Examination of the tumor cells in the stomach revealed that they carried antigens of the P blood group system (or at least an antigen designated Tj^a) that interacted strongly with the anti-P + P_1 + P^k present in her plasma. Thus it seems that the tumor cells, due to their abnormal genome, were able to synthesize P1 system antigens, which were not present upon her red cells. It is concluded that the interaction between the P system antigens on the tumor cells and the antibody in plasma might have been effective in killing nests of metastatic cells derived from the primary growth—in other words, that the plasma antibody was cytotoxic with respect to the tumor cells and prevented subsequent progress of metastatic disease. This is an interesting observation, and since similar examples of spurious antigen formation by tumor cells have been recognized in other blood group systems, it will be interesting to bear in mind the possibility that patients carrying antibodies corresponding to such antigens in their plasma might derive some benefit if those antibodies are cytotoxic to the tumor cells bearing the corresponding antigen.

Anti-P + P_1 + P^k and Spontaneous Abortion

Early reports[33,34] suggested that women of the p phenotype with the anti-P + P_1 + P^k antibody in their plasma had a statistically significant higher rate of spontaneous abortion than that of the general population. Moreover, it seemed that most of the surviving children of such mothers had P1-negative red cells, suggesting that such children who did not inherit a P^{Jk} gene from their fathers were more likely to survive in these circumstances. Later reports[35] tended to contradict this finding.

Some cases of an antibody resembling anti-P + P_1 + P^k occur in women of phenotypes other than p.[36] The antibody, an apparent hemolysin, occurred only transiently among Australian women whose obstetric histories reflected frequent spontaneous abortions. The antibody did not seem to occur, however, in women elsewhere with similar histories. An adequate explanation for this phenomenon has not been forthcoming, although environmental factors present among the Australian population studied might conceivably be involved.

Paroxysmal Cold Hemoglobinuria and Auto-Anti-P (Donath-Landsteiner Antibody)

In 1904 Donath and Landsteiner described a hemolysin that could be induced to attach itself to virtually all red cells at reduced temperatures and would bring about lysis of those cells when rewarmed to 37 C in the presence of serum.[37] This formed the basis for the so-called "Donath-Landsteiner" reaction. For many years, it was thought that the biphasic hemolysin responsible for this phenomenon was a nonspecific entity reacting uniformly with all red cells that were exposed to it. More recently, however, it has been shown uniformly to be an example of a cold-reacting IgG antibody with a specific affinity for the P antigen. Thus, it does not react with red cells of the P_1k, P_2k or p phenotypes.[38-40]

Clinically, the antibody is responsible for an acute form of paroxysmal cold hemoglobinuria (PCH), most typically occurring in children under the age of 14, of equal incidence in both sexes. Typically, there is a history of a flu-like syndrome and/or respiratory infection preceding the attack of hemolysis by some 2 weeks. Inappropriate exposure of the child to cold, particularly where significant chilling occurs due to wearing of inadequate clothing out of doors, results in significant cooling of the blood percolating through the superficial microcirculation. This is sufficient to permit attachment of the autoanti-P antibody to P receptors on the red cells. On returning to a warm environment, binding and activation of complement by the immune complex formed in the cold takes place, and intravascular hemolysis—often of severe and even life-threatening degree—takes place. The attack is frequently associated with a sharp rise in temperature, shaking chills and massive hemoglobinuria. Very considerable destruction of circulating red cells may cause a precipitous fall in hematocrit with all the attendant complications of intravascular red cell destruction. In such cases, transfusion may be essential as a life-saving measure. Theoretically, transfusion with P^k or p red cells should be safe, but the availability of such cells is virtually nonexistent. Where transfusion is a matter of necessity, regular P-positive red cells can be cautiously transfused, the units having been prewarmed to 37 C and delivered to the patient through a blood warmer at 37 C. The patient should be kept thoroughly warm at all times. Suppression of antibody production by the empirical use of steroids is also recommended.[41]

The origin of the Donath-Landsteiner antibody in these cases is probably an immune response to a P-like antigen carried by certain viruses. Generally, antibody titer falls rapidly after recovery from infection and is likely soon to disappear from the circulation.[38,41]

The P Blood Group System and Urinary Tract Infections

Since 1973, a reciprocal relationship between P1-like receptors on the fimbriae of certain strains of *Escherichia coli* and P system receptors on uroepithelial cells in humans has been recognized.[11,41,42] These observations also indicated that young girls who had inherited a P^1 gene (P^{1k}) were more susceptible to urinary tract infections with certain strains of *E. coli* than those who had not. Similarly, it has been shown that persons of the p phenotype are not susceptible to acute pyelonephritis related to certain pyelonephritogenic strains of *E. coli*.[43] In the establishment of urinary tract infections, the short urethra of the female is clearly a significant factor in permitting the entry of organisms into the bladder. The organisms may then secure themselves by preferential attachment to specific receptors on the surface of the uroepithelium of the bladder. This facilitates the progress of the organisms across the surface of the uroepithelium in a ladder-like fashion, which, because of their adherence to the surface, enables them more easily to progress upwards (against the downward urinary flow from the bladder to the ureter) in some cases, to the renal pelvis, where pyelonephritis may become established. The receptors involved appear to possess a projecting terminal D-galactose joined through an $\alpha(1\rightarrow 4)$ linkage to another galactose, these units forming the terminal pair of sugars in a glycosphingolipid oligosaccharide structure located on the uroepithelial cell membrane. This arrangement thus corresponds to P^k or P1 antigenic specificities. Attachment between these structures and corresponding receptors on the fimbriae of the pyelonephritogenic strains of *E. coli* confers an advantage on the organism for upstream progression and for an assault on the kidney. People of p phenotype who do not possess P^k or P1 receptors on uroepithelium would thus have a genetic advantage in resisting such infections over persons of other P1 system phenotypes.[43,44] The receptors on the fimbriae of certain strains of *E. coli* appear to comprise P1-like structures.

Conclusion

Although from the clinical perspective P1 (003) is a system of relatively minor importance, it nonetheless exhibits some features of singular interest. Not the least of these is the role played by P system antigenic determinants in the pathogenesis of pyelonephritis—a disease with significant morbidity and mortality that frequently becomes established in young female children as a relatively asymptomatic disorder. It may ultimately progress to bring about significant destruction of kidney substance and renal function, leading to the disability and death of the patient. From an immunohematologic perspective, the interrelationships between this system and the ABO (001), H (018) and Lewis (007) systems as well as the I (207001) and i (207002) antigens, is illustrative of the ubiquity of blood group glycolipid antigens and of the occurrence of analogous substances in a wide range of species from viruses to humans. The provocations of autoanti-P by viral antigens with major consequences for humans in which this occurs is another case in point.

References

1. Landsteiner K, Levine P. Further observations on individual differences of human blood. Proc Soc Exp Biol Med 1927;24:941-2.
2. Landsteiner K, Levine P. On inheritance and racial distribution of agglutinable properties of human blood. J Immunol 1930;18:87-94.
3. Sanger R. An association between the P and Jay systems of blood groups. Nature 1955;176(4494):1163-4.
4. Issitt PD. The P blood group system. In: Issitt PD, ed. Applied blood group serology. 3rd ed. Miami, FL: Montgomery Scientific Publications, 1985:203-18.
5. Matson GA, Swanson J, Noades J, et al. A new antigen and antibody belonging to the P blood group system. Am J Hum Genet 1959;11(1): 26-34.
6. Lewis M, Anstee DA, Bird GWG, et al. Blood group terminology 1990. From the ISBT working party on terminology for red cell surface antigens. Vox Sang 1990;58:154-69.
7. Raik E, Hunter E, Warner H. Anti-P_1 antibody production after the Casoni skin test. Med J Aust 1970;1(21)1055-7.
8. Marsh WL, Øyen R. A study of soluble Lewis and P_1 substances produced for use in immunohematology. Transfusion 1978;18(6): 743-6.

9. Ben-Ismail R, Rouger P, Carme B, et al. Comparative automated assay of anti-P_1 antibodies in acute hepatic distomiasis (fascioliasis) and in hydatidosis. Vox Sang 1980;38(3):165-8.
10. Nakajima H, Yokota T. Two Japanese families with P^k members. Vox Sang 1977;32(1):56-8.
11. Anstall HB. ABH antigens in disease. In: Wallace ME, Gibbs FR, eds. Blood group systems: ABH and Lewis. Arlington, VA: American Association of Blood Banks, 1986: 135-55.
12. Gill CJ. Structural basis of immunogenicity and antigenic reactivity. In: Ball CA, ed. A seminar on antigen on blood cells and body fluids. Washington, DC: American Association of Blood Banks, 1980:25-33.
13. Watkins WM, Morgan WT. Immunochemical observations on the human blood group P system. J Immunogenet 1976;3(1):15-27.
14. Fellous M, Gerbal A, Tessier C, et al. Studies on the biosynthetic pathway of human P erythrocyte antigens using somatic cells in culture. Vox Sang 1974;26(6):518-36.
15. Naiki M, Marcus DM. An immunochemical study of the human blood group P1, P and P^k glycosphingolipid antigens. Biochemistry 1975; 14(22):4837-41.
16. Marcus DM, Schwarting GA. Immunochemical properties of glycolipids and phospholipids. Adv Immunol 1976;23:203-40.
17. Engelfriet CP, Beckers D, von dem Borne AEGKr, et al. Haemolysins probably recognizing the antigen p. Vox Sang 1972;23(3):176-81.
18. Issitt CH, Duckett JB, Osborne BM, et al. Another example of an antibody reacting optimally with p red cells. Br J Haematol 1976; 34(1):19-23.
19. Crawford MN, Tippett P, Sanger R. Antigens Au^a, i and P1 of cells of the dominant type of Lu(a–b–). Vox Sang 1974;26(3):283-7.
20. Crawford MN, Greenwalt TJ, Saski T, et al. The phenotype Lu(a–b–) together with unconventional Kidd groups in one family. Transfusion 1961;1:228-32.
21. Tippett P, Sanger R, Race RR, et al. An agglutinin associated with the P and the ABO blood group systems. Vox Sang 1965;10:269-80.
22. Adinolfi M, Polley MJ, Hunter DA, Mollison PL. Classification of blood-group antibodies as β2M or gamma globulin. Immunology 1962;5:566-79.
23. Iseki S, Masaki S, Levine P. A remarkable family with the rare human isoantibody anti Tj^a in four siblings: Anti Tj^a and habitual abortion. Nature 1954;173(4416):1192-3.
24. Allen FH Jr, Marsh WL, Jensen L, Fink J. Anti-IP: An antibody defining another product of interaction between the genes of the I and P blood group systems. Vox Sang 1974;27(5):422-6.
25. Booth PB. Anti $I^T P_1$: An antibody showing a further association between the I and P blood group systems. Vox Sang 1970;19(1):85-90.
26. McGinniss MH, Kaplan HS, Bowen AB, Schmidt PJ. Agglutinins for "null" red blood cells. Transfusion 1969;9(1):40-2.

27. Mollison PL, Cutbush M. Use of isotope-labelled red cells to demonstrate incompatibility in vivo. Lancet 1955;268(6878):1290-5.
28. Mollison PL. Factors determining the relative clinical importance of different blood-group antibodies. Br Med Bull 1959;15(2):92-8.
29. Giblett ER. Blood group alloantibodies: An assessment of some laboratory practices. Transfusion 1977;17(4):299-308.
30. Morel PA, Garratty G, Perkins HA. Clinically significant and insignificant antibodies in blood transfusion. Am J Med Technol 1978;44(2):122-9.
31. Vos GH. A comparative observation of the presence of anti-Tj^a-like hemolysins in relation to obstetric history, distribution of the various blood groups and the occurrence of immune anti-A or anti-B hemolysins among aborters and nonaborters. Transfusion 1965;5:327-35.
32. Prokop O, Schlesinger D. Über das Vorkommen von P_1-blutgruppensubstanz oder einer "P_1-like-substance" bei lumbricus Terrestris. Acta Biol Med German 1965;15:180-1.
33. Ahrons S, Kissmeyer-Nielsen F. Febrile transfusion reaction caused by minor specific (LA1) leucocyte incompatibility. A case. Dan Med Bull 1968;15(9):257-8.
34. Levene C, Sela R, Rudolphson Y, et al. Hemolytic disease of the newborn due to anti-PP$_1$P^k (anti-Tj^a). Transfusion 1977;17(6):568-72.
35. Sanger R, Tippett P. Live children and abortion of p mothers (letter). Transfusion 1979;19(2):222-4.
36. Vox GH. A study related to the significance of hemolysins observed among aborters, nonaborters and infertility patients. Transfusion 1967;7(1):40-7.
37. Donath J, Landsteiner K. Über paroxysmale Hämoglobinurie. Münch med Wochenschr 1904;51:1590-3.
38. Levine P, Celano MJ, Falkowski F. The specificity of the antibody in paroxysmal cold hemoglobinuria (PCH). Transfusion 1963;3:278-80.
39. Worlledge SM, Rousso C. Studies on the serology of paroxysmal cold haemoglobinuria (PCH), with special reference to its relationship with the P blood group system. Vox Sang 1965;10:293-8.
40. van der Hart M, van der Giessen M, van der Veer M, et al. Immunochemical and serological properties of biphasic haemolysins. Vox Sang 1964;9:36-9.
41. Anstall HB, Urie PM. Transfusion therapy in special clinical situations. In: Anstall HB, Urie PM. A manual of hemotherapy. New York: John Wiley & Sons, 1986:267-308.
42. Leffler H, Svanborg-Eden C. Glycolipid receptors for uropathogenic receptors *Escherichia coli* on human erythrocytes on uroepithelial cells. Infect Immun 1981;34:920-9.
43. Reid MS, Bird GWG. Associations between human red cell blood group antigens and disease. Transf Med Rev 1990:47-55.

44. MiKush VA. Mendelian inheritance in man. Catalogs of autosomal dominant, autosomol recessive, and X-linked phenotypes. 7th ed. Baltimore, MD: The John Hopkins University Press, 1986.

In: Moulds JM and Woods LL, eds.
Blood Groups: P, I, Sd^a and Pr
Arlington, VA: American Association of Blood Banks, 1991

2

The I Blood Group Collection

Malcolm L. Beck, FIMLS, MIBiol

COLD AGGLUTININS HAVE BEDEVILED and bewildered blood group serologists ever since sera and red cells were mixed together as a preliminary to blood transfusion. Encountered in sera from healthy blood donors as well as in patients suffering from acquired hemolytic anemia, cold agglutinins are IgM autoantibodies that best agglutinate red cells at low temperatures. Agglutinating activity falls dramatically as temperature increases, so that an antibody capable of causing complete agglutination at 4 C may be devoid of activity at 22 C. The molecular basis of this temperature-dependent hemagglutination is unclear.

For many years, cold-reactive antibodies were thought to bind to an antigen common to all human red cells. The term "nonspecific cold agglutinin" was frequently used. Then, in 1956, Wiener et al[1] reported that five donors had been found whose red cells failed to react with a potent "nonspecific cold agglutinin." Such nonreactive donors were very rare. The authors had to test 22,000 New York blood donors to find the five. Wiener and colleagues gave the name I to the antigen detected by their patient's serum. (The I designation was chosen to reflect the individuality of those who lacked the antigen.) Wiener's work thus established the first specificity for cold agglutinins.

With the finding of anti-i by Marsh and colleagues,[2] the specificity loop appeared to close; however, subsequent serologic observations dispelled notions of simplicity and provided hints of the complexity soon to be revealed. Before long, it was clear that a serologic labyrinth existed. Antibodies with great serologic diversity were encountered, leading to the proposal of a mosaic structure of Ii blood groups. To complicate matters further, the Ii blood group antigens refused to be confined within the boundaries of a single system. Borders were not respected—the Ii "sys-

---

Malcolm L. Beck, FIMLS, MIBiol, Technical Director, Community Blood Center of Greater Kansas City, Kansas City, Missouri

tem" was seen trespassing on the turf of ABH, Lewis and P. This serologic complexity could only be explained in terms of antibodies to compound antigens. The logic of chemistry demanded that the appellation "blood group system" be dropped. Recently, the ISBT Working Party on Terminology for Red Cell Surface Antigens has designated Ii as a blood group collection and given it the number 207. Thus, I is 207001 and i is 207002, while other antigens in this group have not yet been assigned numbers.[3]

Serologic History

I and i

The first steps toward establishing the specificity of cold agglutinins were taken in New York in 1956. Wiener and coworkers[1] tested the red cells of 22,000 blood donors with a powerful cold-reacting antibody from a patient with cold antibody hemolytic anemia. The red cells of five blood donors that failed to react with this antibody were said to lack a very common antigen designated I. It was thought that these nonreactors must be homozygous for a very rare gene responsible for producing the antigen i, although no data from family studies were available to support this hypothesis.

Four years later, on the other side of the Atlantic, the next significant steps toward increasing our understanding of the Ii blood groups were taken. In 1960, Jenkins et al[4] described the red cells of Mr. M, a healthy blood donor to the Regional Blood Transfusion Center, Brentwood, England. Mr. M's blood sample distinguished itself as an ABO blood grouping problem: the red cells appeared to be group A, whereas the serum gave the reactions expected of group O. The cause of this anomaly was a potent cold agglutinin. Unexpectedly, Mr. M's cold agglutinin was not an autoantibody. The alert minds in Brentwood were soon on the track of a new specificity. The red cells and serum of Mr. M were systematically tested with all ABO-compatible samples referred to the Brentwood consultation laboratory. About 1 year (and many samples) later, this endeavor was rewarded when Mr. M's cells failed to react with the serum of a patient referred by the London Chest Hospital. The patient had acute hemolytic anemia associated with a potent, high-titer cold autoagglutinin similar to that with which Wiener had defined the I antigen in New York. Sera from five other patients with cold antibody hemolytic anemia, as well as 50 sera containing nonspecific cold agglutinins, were also found to react only very weakly with Mr. M's cells. It was concluded that the patients' antibodies were anti-I and that Mr. M's red cells must lack the I antigen. A search of 17,000 other blood donors failed to disclose another example of the i phenotype; however, it was observed that cells of newborns were nonreactive or only very weakly reactive with anti-I. (See Table 2-1.)

Table 2-1. Typical Reactions of Anti-I at 4 C

Dilutions	2	4	8	16	32	64	128
Group O adult	4+	4+	3+	2+	1	0	0
Group O cord	1+	±	0	0	0	0	0

Two conclusions could be drawn from these studies. The first was that nearly all cold-reactive autoagglutinins had I specificity. The second, and most significant, was that although variable reactivity was noted with different anti-I sera,[2,5] the I antigen was very weakly expressed on cord cells.[4] This second conclusion subsequently permitted easy recognition of anti-I by inclusion of cord blood cells in antibody identification panels.

Marsh and colleagues encountered another cold autoantibody, with some atypical serologic characteristics, about a year later. The patient had severe autoimmune hemolytic anemia secondary to reticulum cell sarcoma. The intriguing feature of this case was that severe hemolysis was associated with a relatively modest cold autoagglutinin. When titrated against red cells from normal adults, the titer did not exceed 16. The true nature of this "new" antibody became apparent when titration studies with cord cells revealed a titer of 200,000! Ever mindful of "carry-over" in serial dilution procedures, Marsh and colleagues prepared absolute dilutions of 1 in 50,000 and 1 in 100,000. Each dilution gave strong reactions with i adult cells at 12 C. The reactivity of this new antibody was seen to be virtually antithetical to that expected of anti-I, and an article by Marsh and Jenkins entitled "Anti-i: a new cold antibody" soon appeared in *Nature*.[2]

For a 3-year period Mr. M's red cells were used to screen the sera of 500 normal donors as well as all reference samples containing cold-reactive antibodies. Only two other examples of anti-i were found: one in a fatal case of hemolytic anemia complicating an obscure malignant reticulosis, and the other in a young woman with infectious mononucleosis.[6] Shortly after this study, a fourth example of anti-i was observed, again associated with hemolytic anemia complicating infectious mononucleosis.[7] Anti-i was obviously very rarely produced; however, the finding that two of four examples were associated with infectious mononucleosis pointed the way to a much richer source.

Change in Ii Antigens With Age

Race and Sanger[8] demonstrated that whereas red cell I antigen expression varies considerably from one donor to another, in any given individual the expression remains relatively constant. After Jenkins et al[4] showed that the I antigen on cord cells was very poorly developed, Marsh[6] studied the red cells of 62 normal infants and children ranging in age from 2 days up to 4 years. Using serial titrations he demonstrated that while cord cells are rich in i antigen, over the first 18 months of life i antigen is gradually lost as I is gained in a reciprocal relationship.

The foundations for understanding the Ii blood groups at the serologic level were thus firmly established. The common cold autoagglutinins found often in normal sera, as well as the pathologic cold autoantibody causing hemolytic anemia, were shown to have I specificity, although their other serologic characteristics were strikingly different. Rarely encountered were examples of a cold agglutinin that reacted strongly with the red cells of adults lacking the I antigen (i adult). These sera were said to have specificity for the i antigen.[2,6] Using potent anti-I and anti-i reagents, Marsh[6] concluded that all cells possessed both I and i, in a somewhat antithetical relationship. Normal adult cells were rich in I, but possessed at least trace amounts of i. Cord cells and adult cells of the very rare i phenotype possessed abundant i receptors, but only scant amounts of I.

Serologic Heterogeneity of Ii Blood Groups

Early in the investigation of the Ii blood groups, Marsh[2] and Tippett[5] encountered some examples of cold agglutinins that appeared to have specificity directed at ABH-Ii complexes and other examples that seemed to be directed toward I subgroups. Evidence of considerable heterogeneity accumulated and a series of Ii-related subspecificities and complex specificities were proposed. The age of simplicity had passed quickly.

Subspecificities

I^T

In 1965, Curtain and colleagues[9] reported a high incidence of cold agglutinins in sera of the Kuanua people of New Britain, Melanesia. In addition to the high frequency of these cold agglutinins, the majority (39/45) did not demonstrate simple anti-I specificity when tested with cord cells and adult cells. The authors considered it likely that these antibodies were directed toward an undetermined high-incidence antigen.

Booth and coworkers[10] confirmed the high incidence of cold autoagglutinins in Melanesian sera, and carried out detailed serologic investigations on six of these. Although one reacted as anti-I, results of titration studies (against I adult, i adult and cord cells) on the other five sera were not typical of anti-I or anti-i. These sera reacted weakly with I adult and i adult cells, but reacted strongly with cord cells. Red cells of Cynamolgus monkeys, known to be rich in i antigen, were also only weakly reactive.

Adsorption and elution studies demonstrated the presence of a single antibody specificity directed against a component of the Ii antigens not previously defined. The weak reactions observed with i-adult and Cynamolgus monkey cells established that the sera did not have simple i specificity. Similarly, the weak reactions with normal adult cells militated against I specificity. Nevertheless, weak reactions with i adult cells strongly supported a relationship to I. The strong reactions with cord cells and the weak reactions with i adult cells suggested that the antibody was directed against a part of the I antigen in the process of development. This I antigen subdeterminant was present in maximum amount on cord cells during the normal transition from i to I. The term I^T was adopted to recognize the antigen's transitional nature.

Booth[11] later suggested that I^T might not represent a transitional state because he found Melanesians with reduced levels of I^T, but apparently normal amounts of I and i. Garratty et al[12] supported Booth's initial view with the observation that I^T is strongly expressed on fetal cells.

In 1968, Layrisse and Layrisse[13] reported that 84% of sera from Yanomama Indians of Venezuela contained anti-I^T as a cold autoagglutinin. A later investigation of Venezuelan populations by these authors[14] confirmed the previous observations in Yanomama Indians and extended them to include other Indian populations within the same limited geographic area. In the case of the Venezuelan studies, I^T specificity was established by showing little difference in titration endpoints between adult and cord red cells. Differences amounting to less than two dilutions were considered as indicative of anti-I^T specificity. This definition of I^T is not precisely the same as that given by Booth et al[10]; they defined anti-I^T as reacting weakly with I adult and i adult, but strongly with cord cells. Layrisse assigned I^T specificity to sera that reacted with both adult and cord cells and to a lesser extent with Rhesus monkey cells (which are rich in i). The differences in the titration endpoints reported by Layrisse are not entirely persuasive. For example, one representative serum was reportedly reactive with cord cells, normal adult cells and Rhesus monkey cells to titers of 256, 128 and 64 respectively.[13] Such differences in titer might be regarded as too small to define I^T specificity with confidence. (See Table 2-2.)

Other cold antibody specificities revealed in the Layrisse study were equally unexpected. It was reported that anti-i was present in 14% of Yanomamas and in 4% of healthy Caracas blood donors.[13] The inconsistencies of antibody frequencies reported by different workers were perhaps

Table 2-2. Typical Reactions of Anti-I^T at 4 C

Dilutions	2	4	8	16	32	64	128
I adult	3+	3+	2+	1+	0	0	0
i adult	2+	1+	±	±	0	0	0
Cord	3+	3+	3+	2+	1+	±	0

a prelude to the serologic complexity revealed with the unfolding story of the Ii blood groups.

Inhibitable and Noninhibitable Anti-I

In 1970, Dzierzkowa-Borodej et al[15] described an inhibitable anti-I. This was a novel finding; previously, examples of anti-I had not proved to be inhibitable.[6] Inhibition was observed with hydatid cyst fluid, saliva and human milk. Using milk as a source of I substance, Marsh et al[16] showed that among 24 anti-I sera, inhibition was quite variable and easily inhibitable anti-I sera were rare. In sum, these studies suggested that at least two kinds of anti-I existed: inhibitable and noninhibitable.

I^D and I^F

At this point (1971), it was evident that Ii blood groups were a heterogeneous complex of epitopes reflecting fine biochemical structural differences. Convinced that the I antigen was of a mosaic nature, Marsh and colleagues[17] proposed the terms I^D and I^F to designate two subdeterminants that could be identified serologically.

It was recognized that even cord cells possessed some expression of I. I^D was described as that part of the I mosaic that was absent or very poorly developed on cord cells. I^D was gradually acquired (at the expense of i) during the first 18 months of life, and was fully expressed on adult cells. Cord cells were thought to possess a part of the I mosaic distinct from I^D. To reflect the fetal origins of this part of the I mosaic, it was given the name I^F. I^F was considered to be fundamental to all human red cells, including i adults. The expression of I^F appeared to be stable and not subject to developmental maturity over the first months of life. The small amount of I antigen on Rhesus monkey red cells was thought to be of the I^F type. Anti-I sera that gave relatively strong reactions with i adult cells and cord cells were considered to be anti-I^F.

I^S

Some sera with anti-I activity could be neutralized by human colostrum or milk as well as by saliva.[18] The soluble substance with I activity was called I^S. Presumably, those examples of anti-I^D that were found by Marsh et al[16] to be inhibitable would be classified as anti-I^S by Dzierzkowa-Borodej.

With the advantage of hindsight, it may seem to the reader (as it does to this reviewer) that it is risky to assign subspecificities within a system notable for a wide range of phenotypic expression. On the other hand, when biochemical data are not available to clarify perceived serologic specificities, assigned names may facilitate communication.

Complexes of I, ABH and P

During the early studies of the Ii blood groups, Marsh observed that the activity of some anti-I sera was influenced by the ABO group of the test cells. As early as 1960 Tippett,[5] with great perception, noted, "It may be that the substance which the I genes are stamping with specificity is connected with one of the steps that lead to the formation of the ABO antigens." In the light of current knowledge of the biochemical relationship of the Ii and ABO systems, it is not surprising that I "system" antibodies might have a complex specificity.

IA

An antibody that reacted preferentially with cells carrying both I and A was described by Tippett in 1960.[5] The serum failed to react with group A i adult cells and with group O I adult cells. It reacted more strongly with A_1I cells than with A_2I cells. The antibody, dubbed anti-IA, appeared to be directed toward a compound of antigens A and I. The antibody did not react with Ai cells and was not inhibited by A secretor saliva. In 1964, a serum with the same specificity was reported by Gold,[19] along with accounts of other sera displaying compound specificities. Reports of additional examples followed thick and fast. Melanesia proved to be an exceedingly rich source of antibodies to compound antigens.[20,21] Numerous examples of anti-IA have since been encountered. (See Table 2-3.)

IB

The first reports of an antibody requiring the presence of both I and B antigens came from Salmon and colleagues[22] and from Tegoli et al.[23]

Table 2-3. Typical Reactions of Anti-IA at 4 C

Dilutions	1	2	4	8	16
AI adult	4+	3+	3+	1+	0
Ai adult	1+	±	0	0	0
A cord	1+	0	0	0	0
OI adult	2+	±	0	0	0

Salmon reported cases of hemolytic anemia in which red cell eluate specificities included examples of anti-IA, -IB and -IH. (Objections to the anti-IB specificities have been raised because group O cells could adsorb the anti-IB activity.[24]) Tegoli and coworkers[23] reported the finding of a cold autoagglutinin in the serum of a group B patient with carcinoma. This antibody reacted preferentially with cells positive for both I and B.

Drachmann[25] described a group AB patient whose serum contained a cold agglutinin that had a special affinity for cells possessing I and B. Cord cells belonging to groups O, A and B were nonreactive. The anti-IB activity could be abolished by group B and A_2B secretor saliva, unlike the antibody described by Tegoli et al.[23] Titration scores demonstrated greater activity with A_2B and B than with A_1B cells. The author preferred the term anti-BI(O) to reflect the additional H affinity. This antibody appears to define an epitope constructed by products of the *H*, *I* and *B* genes.

A further example of anti-IB causing anomalous compatibility testing results was reported by Morel and coworkers in 1975.[26] The patient was group B, but his serum proved to be incompatible with group B units at room temperature. Group O reagent red cells, the patient's own group B cells and group B cord cells were not agglutinated. This antibody was not inhibited by group O or B secretor saliva or by human milk. In studies at 4 C, the patient's own cells and all other group B cells were strongly agglutinated; group O adult cells reacted weakly, group B cord cells reacted very weakly and group O cord cells reacted not at all. This antibody was not detectable 1 month later. The authors concluded that the patient's serum contained anti-IB. In a deliberate search for anti-IB, Voak et al[24] studied a series of normal group A sera. By absorption and neutralization procedures, they demonstrated the fairly frequent occurrence of an anti-IB component. (See Table 2-4.)

IH, H(i) and O(i)

Anti-H was thought to be quite common in sera from A_1 and A_1B subjects until Rosenfield et al[27] demonstrated that, in many cases, agglutinating activity was restricted to cells possessing both I and H antigens. Anti-IH now appears to be the most frequently encountered antibody recognizing a compound antigen of the Ii ABH complex. A related surprise was the

Table 2-4. Typical Reactions of Anti-IB at 4 C

Dilutions	1	2	4	8	16
BI adult	2+	2+	1+	±	0
OI adult	±	±	0	0	0
B cord	1+	0	0	0	0

report of Marcus et al[28] that the degree and rate of inactivation of I antigen by various enzyme preparations was influenced by the ABO group. The I antigen on group A_1 was more rapidly and completely inactivated than I on group O cells.

Rosenfield[27] studied 12 sera containing cold agglutinins with the serologic characteristics of anti-H. None reacted with group Oi adult cells or with group O cord cells or with Oh cells. Rosenfield designated the specificity of 11 of these sera as IH. The 12th, which was inhibitable by H substance, was called anti-H(-i). Schmidt and McGinniss[29] also observed IH-related specificities and commented on the inhibitable specificity H(-i), which they referred to as O(-i).

A cold agglutinin with unusual specificity was found in the serum of a 15-year-old Chinese boy by Giblett et al.[30] The cold agglutinin resembled anti-IH except that it reacted strongly with Oh cells and to some extent with any cell possessing either H or I. The weakest reacting cells were deficient in both I and H. Attempts to separate this cold agglutinin into two specificities were not successful. Lodge and Voak[31] described an example of anti-IH that reacted weakly with group A_2 adult cells, but not with group B adult cells, despite the similar H status of these phenotypes. Steric hindrance by the B antigen was proposed to explain these observations.

iH

Bird and Wingham[32] described a cold agglutinin in the serum of an 80-year-old woman with a pancreatic cyst. The antibody was only very weakly reactive with the patient's own and other group A_1 cells. Strong reactions with A_2i cells and negative reactions with Oh cells argued against IH specificity. The antibody's strong reactions with group O and A_2 cells suggested anti-H; however, the much stronger activity with A_2i cells (as compared with A_2I cells) indicated that specificity was actually directed toward i and H. The paucity of other reports suggested that this was a very rare specificity. In 1990, Pierce and colleagues[33] recognized that without the use of A_2i cells, further examples would masquerade as anti-H. These authors added three more cases to the literature. (See Table 2-5.)

Table 2-5. Typical Reactions of Anti-iH

Dilutions	1	2	4	8	16	32
OI adult	3+	3+	2+	1+	0	0
O cord	4+	4+	4+	3+	2+	1+
Oi adult	4+	3+	3+	2+	2+	1+
A_1i adult	2+	1+	0	0	0	0
A_2i adult	3+ s	3+ s	3+	1+	0	0

IP_1

In 1968, Issitt et al[34] described a new (but expected) specificity, anti-IP_1. Anti-IP_1 agglutinated red cells that were both I and P1 positive. A practical application of this discovery was that anti-P1 reagents composed predominantly of anti-IP_1 could not be relied upon to determine the P_1 type of cord blood samples. Anti-IP_1 was not neutralized by hydatid cyst fluid. Booth[35] described anti-I^TP_1 in 1970. Anti-I^TP_1 is presumably the Melanesian equivalent of anti-IP_1. The antibody was detected in a Melanesian man suffering from hypersplenism. Anti-I^TP_1 failed to react with adult P_1- red cells and was not inhibited by hydatid cyst fluid.

ILe^{bH}

A new antibody specificity, anti-ILe^{bH}, was identified by Tegoli et al[36] in the serum of a 55-year-old woman with terminal carcinoma of the bladder. The antibody reacted only with group O or A_2 I, Le(a–b+) red cells. Saliva containing I, H and Le^b was inhibitory.

Genetics and Biochemistry

The Genetic Basis of the Ii Blood Groups

The precise genetic basis of the Ii blood groups is not known. Although Marsh[6] demonstrated a reciprocal relationship between I and i antigens during the first year of life, there is no evidence that the genes associated with Ii antigenic activity are alleles. A further complication resides in the observations of excessive numbers of i sibs in informative families. It seems likely that the product of the *I* gene is a transferase enzyme involved in the biosynthetic pathways leading to the ABO and P systems. Individuals who are i adult may be homozygous for a very rare amorphic gene.

The Biochemical Basis of the Ii Blood Groups

In recent years, much has been learned about the nature of blood group antigens through a combination of serologic, genetic and biochemical studies. The Ii blood groups provide an excellent example of serologic observations finding a very satisfying biochemical explanation. It is now known that a linear oligosaccharide containing repeating N-acetyllactosamine residues defines i activity. The I antigen is a branched oligosaccharide elaborated from the same linear structures.

Clues to the biochemical structure of the Ii receptors came from early serologic observations. Antibodies with complex specificities involving

ABH as well as Ii pointed strongly to a close relationship to ABH and, therefore, to carbohydrate receptors. Largely due to early work by Feizi, Hakomori, Watanabe and Kabat (reviewed elsewhere[37,38]), it is now clear that the Ii antigens are internal precursor structures in the biosynthetic pathways leading to the ABH determinants. Biochemical knowledge of the ABH glycoconjugates paved the way to an understanding of the nature of the Ii receptors on red cells when Ii-active glycolipid material was successfully isolated.

The ABH determinants on red cells are glycoconjugates composed of oligosaccharides linked to proteins (glycoproteins) and to lipids (glycosphingolipids). Because Ii determinants reside in the ABH core structures, it follows that they too must be expressed on glycoproteins and glycolipids.

It has been estimated that about 75% of red-cell-bound ABO antigens are carried on glycoproteins; the remaining 25% are on glycolipids. The glycoprotein-associated ABH antigens are complex structures based on polylactosamines located on bands 3 and 4.5.[38] Each red cell possesses about one million and 0.5 million monomers of bands 3 and 4.5, respectively. It is highly probable that other, less abundant glycoproteins also possess ABH activity. ABO antigens also occur on a variety of glycolipids. Approximately 0.5 million poly-N-acetyllactosaminyl glycolipids are located in the red cell membrane. Anstee estimated the total number of potential ABH (and therefore Ii) sites to exceed two million per red cell.[39]

The ABH determinants synthesized on red cells are carried predominantly on oligosaccharide precursor chains of the Type 2 variety. Various core structures, which compose these Type 2 chains, give rise to four different H-active chains: H_1, H_2, H_3 and H_4. Blood group Ii activity resides in these core structures and is directly related to the presence of poly-N-acetyllactosamines and the presence or absence of core branching. H_1 and H_2 chains are linear. H_3 and H_4 are branched chains. Nonbranching core structures containing at least two repeating N-acetyllactosamine [Gal β(1→4)GlcNAc] units define i activity. Branched core structures are reactive with anti-I.[40] (See Fig 2-1.)

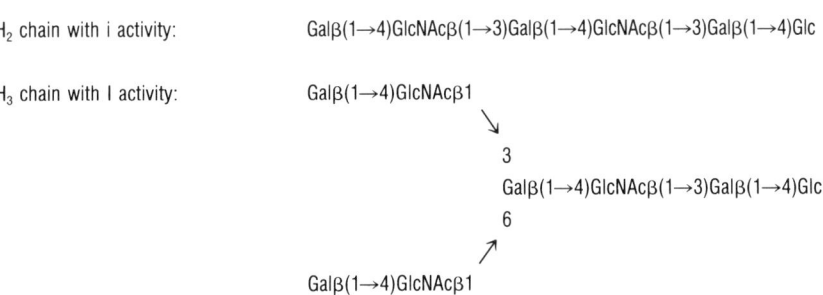

Figure 2-1. Examples of H chains with I and i activity.

Core structures may be "completed" to form H, A and B, may remain "incomplete" or may be sialylated. Fucosylation of the core structure suppresses Ii activity. Incomplete (unsubstituted) and sialylated core structures express Ii activity most fully. H_1 chain cores are devoid of i activity because these short chains do not contain repeating N-acetyllactosamines. H_2 chain cores are linear unbranched structures containing multiple N-acetyllactosamine units; they exhibit i activity. These are the major source of i antigen on red cells.

H_3 and H_4 chain cores are branched oligosaccharides containing repeating N-acetyllactosamine units and displaying I activity. These chains comprise the I antigens on human red cells and are generated after birth by the addition of an N-acetylglucosamine unit in (1→6) linkage to the penultimate galactose residue in the unbranched chain. [Various examples of anti-I are inhibited by structures including the (1→6), the (1→3) or both the (1→6) and (1→3) linked carbohydrate branches.] H_4 chain cores are heterogenous and not well-characterized, but consist of both branched and linear regions. Investigations of rabbit erythrocytes suggest the linear regions may contribute to the sparse i sites demonstrable on adult red cells.[41] It is likely that the product of the I gene is a branching transferase, presumably an $\alpha(1\rightarrow 6)$ glucosaminyltransferase; however, no such enzyme has yet been isolated from the red cell.[42]

The red cells of newborns contain predominantly unbranched linear chains of the H_2 core type and are, therefore, rich in i antigen. Adult red cells are characterized by I-bearing branched chains generated after birth. As expected, a lack of branched oligosaccharides has been demonstrated in the rare adults with the i phenotype. It seems likely that the other subspecificities within the Ii blood groups, (I^F, I^D, I^T, I^S) may represent slight topochemical shifts from one another. Other topochemical relationships between ABH, Ii and P may define the compound antigens. If so, serologic observation will have found a perfect biochemical correlate.

Hemagglutination and the Effect of Temperature on Ii Antigens

The traditional view of cold hemagglutination favored temperature-dependent antibody conformation. It was thought that the antibody changed shape as the temperature increased. This shape change was thought to hinder antibody-antigen complexing. Rosse and Sherwood[43] had a different view; they proposed that temperatures affected conformation of antigen rather than antibody. This proposal was based on observations of antibody affinity changes. According to their argument, temperature-induced changes in antibody conformation should be the same regardless of whether the antibody was reacting with adult or cord cells. However, at higher temperatures actual changes in affinity of antibody for cord cells were greater than those for adult cells. This observation was thought to imply that the conformational changes had taken place, either in the antigen or the cell surface, and to a greater extent on cord cells.

In a later study, Rosse and Lauf[44] demonstrated that solubilized I antigen complexed with anti-I equally as well at 37 C as at 0 C. Moreover, these workers recovered as much I antigen from cord cells as from adult cells. The latter observation is difficult to reconcile with a modern view of the carbohydrate branching characteristics of adult and cord cells. It is also difficult to reconcile with the observation of Gardas and Koscielak,[45] who found that isolated I-active material reacted well at 4 C, but not at all at 37 C.

As mentioned above, Rosse and Lauf[44] proposed that temperature-induced changes of the red cell membrane might be an important feature of cold hemagglutination. They suggested that membrane organization resulted in a receptor that at 37 C was cryptic, but as the temperature dropped toward 0 C, became progressively more available. Later studies of Shinitzky and Soroujon,[46] Borochov and Shinitzky[47] and Basu et al[48] provided evidence that red cell antigenic expression may be modulated by temperature-induced changes of membrane microviscosity. Flamm and colleagues[49] extended these observations to include an investigation of red cell I antigen. These workers suggested that the temperature range of 16-20 C might be a crucial barrier to cold hemagglutination. At temperatures below this range, the membrane lipid may separate into gel-like and fluid-like domains. Preferential partition of the I-reactive components into the fluid regions would increase the local antigen concentration and facilitate antibody-antigen binding at lower temperature.

Pathologic Significance

Cold Hemagglutinin Disease

The Ii blood groups are unique. No red cell, regardless of phenotype, is completely devoid of either antigen, and the defining antibodies are autoantibodies found in the sera of many, if not all, normal healthy individuals.[5,50] Antibody and antigen coexist without evoking the wrath of Ehrlich simply because the thermal range of the antibody activity does not extend to body temperature. This restricted thermal range is the fundamental criterion distinguishing the normal cold autoagglutinin from the pathologic autoantibody. The autoanti-I frequently encountered in blood bank practice reacts only at low temperatures and, therefore, has no significance beyond being a serologic nuisance. In rare cases, however, the thermal amplitude broadens to such an extent that in vivo hemolysis results. This is the basis of cold hemagglutinin disease (CHD), which occurs in two forms: chronic and acute. Chronic CHD results from the persistent production of monoclonal anti-I with elevated thermal amplitude. Acute CHD typically follows mycoplasma or viral infection and is characterized by transient production of polyclonal autoanti-I with high titer and wide thermal range. Hemolysis in acute CHD can be massive, abrupt and, needless to say, alarming.

In CHD a clone of immunocytes producing an antibody with host-destructive tendencies proliferates. Why this is permitted is a question that remains to be answered. It is usual to invoke impairment of T-cell function to account for the failure of self-discrimination. Both decreased suppressor activity and increased helper activity have been proposed; however, it is not clear what is cause and what is effect.

CHD was well-recognized as a clinical entity long before Ii blood group specificity was established.[51] The term nonspecific cold autoagglutinin was frequently used to describe the causative autoantibody. With great foresight, Wiener[52] predicted that a specificity could be assigned to these agglutinins and suspected that it would reside in the nuclear substance of ABH. Three years later he proved that specificity existed after painstakingly testing red cells of 22,000 blood donors with serum from a patient with CHD. When he found five to be nonreactive, it was clear that the nonspecific cold autoagglutinin terminology was inappropriate and Wiener named the antibody anti-I.[1] With the finding of anti-i by Marsh and colleagues[2] and the subsequent observation that cord cells behaved as I negative, it was soon evident that the common cold autoagglutinin found in normal sera also had I specificity. It was also clearly evident that anti-I, as found in normal serum, did not cause in vivo hemolysis.

Typical Benign and Pathogenic Examples of Anti-I

Normal anti-I is an IgM autoagglutinin exhibiting strongest activity at low temperature (0-4 C). It is thought that antibody binding is inversely related to temperature; that is, progressively less antibody is bound as the temperature is increased. As the temperature approaches 37 C, very little or no antibody complexes with the red cell membrane (at least no agglutination occurs). Alloanti-I is found in the serum of most i adults. It reacts best at 0-4 C and rarely is active above room temperature.

Pathologic anti-I is also an IgM autoagglutinin, but has a much broader thermal range and is characteristically far more potent than the benign antibodies described above. Some examples of autoantibodies causing CHD have titers greater than 1×10^6 at 4 C. This increased potency may obscure antibody specificity unless the serum is tested in titration at the upper end of its thermal range against adult and cord cells. Undiluted sera will often react equally well with adult and cord cells, especially at 4 C. The most important differential criterion distinguishing a pathologic anti-I is the increased thermal range of agglutinating activity. When the thermal range of IgM anti-I encompasses body temperature, the patient may develop severe intravascular hemolysis because IgM antibodies are efficient complement activators. (See Table 2-6.)

Table 2-6. Typical Reactions of Anti-I From a Case of Cold Agglutinin Disease

Dilutions	2	4	8	16	32	64	128	256	512	1024	2048	4096
Tests at 4 C												
OI adult	4+	4+	4+	4+	4+	4+	4+	3+	2+	1+	±	0
Oi adult	4+	4+	4+	4+	3+	3+	2+	±	0	0	0	0
Cord	4+	4+	4+	4+	4+	4+	3+	2+	±	0	0	0
Tests at 20 C												
OI adult	4+	4+	4+	3+	1+	1+	0	0	0	0	0	0
Oi adult	2+	1+	0	0	0	0	0	0	0	0	0	0
Cord	2+	2+	±	0	0	0	0	0	0	0	0	0
Tests at 30 C												
OI adult	2+	±	0	0	0	0	0	0	0	0	0	0
Oi adult	0	0	0	0	0	0	0	0	0	0	0	0
Cord	0	0	0	0	0	0	0	0	0	0	0	0
Tests at 37 C												
OI adult	0	0	0	0	0	0	0	0	0	0	0	0
Oi adult	0	0	0	0	0	0	0	0	0	0	0	0
Cord	0	0	0	0	0	0	0	0	0	0	0	0

It is important to note that the thermal range of the autoantibody-induced hemagglutination need not extend to 37 C. In fact, very few cases of CHD are associated with cold antibodies that agglutinate red cells in tests performed strictly at 37 C. Thermal amplitude studies will usually demonstrate no agglutination at temperatures exceeding 30 C. However, in vivo temperatures can be as low as 30-32 C in the peripheral circulation of the patient, especially if the ambient temperature is low. Many patients become symptomatic during cold winter weather when in vivo temperatures, especially in the extremities, will fall within the range of antibody activity. Under these conditions, autoagglutination causes vascular occlusion, giving rise to Raynaud's phenomenon in exposed parts of the body. Although antibody will elute from the red cells as they circulate to warmer parts of the body, complement activation can lead to intravascular hemolysis. Agglutination may not always be a prerequisite of complement activation. Transient contact of antibody with red cells at 37 C may activate complement and lead to hemolysis.[53] This description of the pathogenesis of CHD applies to both chronic (with monoclonal autoantibody production) and acute (with transient, polyclonal antibody production) CHD. Occasionally, other I series antibodies will be incriminated in CHD and, very rarely, autoantibody specificity may be directed to antigens of other blood group systems. The typical case, however, is associated with a wide thermal range, IgM, anti-I autoagglutinin. Petz and Garratty[54] incriminated anti-I in 49 of a series of 54 cases.

Both chronic and acute CHD are treated identically. In essence, this consists of raising the patient's environmental temperature to a level beyond the thermal range of the antibody. Usually, turning up the thermostat controlling the room air temperature and the use of electrically heated blankets are adequate. Most cases can be managed without resorting to blood transfusion. When transfusion is unavoidable, a sufficiently low drip rate should be used so that no appreciable body cooling occurs. In extreme cases a blood warmer may be needed.

Ii Antibodies and Infections

Anti-I and Mycoplasma pneumoniae Infection

Mycoplasma pneumoniae infection has long been associated with an increase in the titer and thermal range of autoanti-I.[55,56] When the antibody's thermal range includes body temperature (as described above), hemolysis can be rapid and alarming in patients otherwise not desperately ill. Ironically, hemolysis may occur just as the infection appears to be resolving. Hemolysis is usually transient and self-limiting, but in extreme cases hemoglobin levels may fall dramatically in a matter of hours. Fatalities attributed to such hemolysis have been recorded.[57,58]

The sera of patients with *M. pneumoniae* infections are characterized by the presence of high titer, high thermal range anti-I. Analysis of light chains shows the presence of both κ and λ, confirming polyclonal origins. It has been proposed that the anti-I produced is primarily in response to a *M. pneumoniae* antigen, but the antibody is cross-reactive with a red cell antigen, presumably I-related.[59] Although intact *M. pneumoniae* organisms do not neutralize anti-I activity, a lipopolysaccharide extract has proved to be inhibitory. Moreover, Costea et al[60] were able to produce cold agglutinins in rabbits by injections of *M. pneumoniae*. Thus, it appears there may be validity in the concept that the increase in anti-I titer associated with *M. pneumoniae* infection can be attributed to an immune response to the organism. Schmidt et al[61] and Feizi,[62] however, suggested that the increase in anti-I titer may represent a response to *Mycoplasma* modified "self" I antigen.

Petz and Garratty[54] pointed out that, whereas only 51 cases of overt immune hemolytic anemia have been reported in the world literature, subclinical hemolysis may be common. One case worthy of special mention was reported by Bell et al.[63] This case report associated *M. pneumoniae* infection with paroxysmal cold hemoglobinuria (PCH) in a 17-year-old boy. The specificity of the biphasic hemolysin was anti-I. I and HI specificity have been associated with PCH only rarely.[64]

Anti-I and Epstein-Barr Virus (EBV)

Cold autoantibody-induced hemolysis is an uncommon complication of infectious mononucleosis. In the majority of cases the autoantibody has i specificity. Although overt hemolysis is infrequent, the occurrence of anti-i in the serum of infectious mononucleosis patients is not. Marsh and Jenkins[2] encountered only three examples of anti-i during a search that lasted 3 years. Notably, the third example was found in a patient with infectious mononucleosis complicated by hemolytic anemia. This observation prompted a study of the incidence of anti-i in patients with infectious mononucleosis.[7] Anti-i was found in 8% of 85 cases in the study. The anti-i was shown to be distinct from the Paul-Bunnell heterophile antibody. In three cases, the anti-i was shown to be composed of IgM. Rosenfield et al[65] embarked on a similar study of 38 sera from cases of infectious mononucleosis. These workers reported that 68% contained anti-i. Worlledge and Dacie[66] reviewed the literature and concluded that, whereas anti-i could be demonstrated in about 50% of cases of infectious mononucleosis, hemolysis occurred in less than 1%. They attributed the variability of the reported incidence of anti-i to the methods used and the population studied. Hoagland[67] reported an incidence of 3%.

Overall, the literature suggests that anti-i is a common cold agglutinin in the sera of patients suffering from infectious mononucleosis. It is IgM, transient, of relatively low titer and of a low thermal range. Horwitz et al[68] studied the cold agglutinins in a variety of patients with various mononucleosis syndromes including both heterophile antibody positive and negative cases. They concluded that anti-i agglutinins were characteristic of EBV infections. Only very rarely, in less than 1% of cases, does the thermal range of the antibody extend to clinically significant temperatures. (In the case reported by Troxel et al[69] the titer of anti-i at 37 C was 128.) In these cases hemolytic episodes can occur. The degree of anemia may be mild to severe. The presence of cold-reactive IgG anti-i complexed with IgM anti-IgG was reported by Goldberg and Barnett[70] and Capra et al,[71] but has not been confirmed by others. A case of infectious mononucleosis and hemolytic anemia was reported by Gronemeyer et al.[72] The patient was found to have a cold-reactive IgG anti-i as well as cold-reactive rheumatoid factor (IgM anti-IgG). In general, it appears that autoimmune hemolysis, complicating infectious mononucleosis, is due to the transient production of IgM autoanti-i; however, the presence of relatively low thermal range antibodies in some cases suggests that a nonimmune mechanism of red cell destruction may also operate.[73] The possibility of a biphasic anti-i hemolysin was raised by Burkart and Hsu.[74]

Cold Autoagglutinins and Other Infections

An increased incidence of high-titered cold agglutinins in patients with influenza A and B infections has been observed. Finland and Barnes[75] reported that 5 of 144 patients developed high-titer cold agglutinins. This incidence is much lower than that reported for either *M. pneumoniae* or EBV infections. Similarly, hemolytic anemia attributed to high-titered cold agglutinins, in cases of infection other than *M. pneumoniae* or EBV, has been reported rarely.[76-79]

A few examples of cold-antibody-induced hemolytic anemia complicating other viral infections have been recorded. These include hemolytic anemia associated with cold autoantibodies in a case of *Coxsackie A* virus infection reported by Betke et al,[80] and a transient increase in anti-I titer documented following an acute cytomegalovirus infection.[81]

Pirofsky[82] has gleaned from the early literature a series of diseases that have been associated with cold agglutinins and hemolytic anemia. These include relapsing fever, malaria, trypanosomiasis and bacterial infections. Increase in cold agglutinin titers associated with malaria and trypanosomiasis was documented by Marienberg.[83] Marienberg demonstrated cold agglutinins in rats, rabbits and guinea pigs following inoculation with trypanosomes. Pirofsky[82] pointed out, however, that the etiologic significance of these relationships may be questionable.

High-titered anti-I has been documented following *Listeria monocytogenes* infection. The infection was associated with hemolytic anemia[84] in a 61-year-old, excessively beer-drinking tailor. Injection of killed *Listeria* organisms produced significant titers of cold agglutinins in rabbits.

Cold Agglutinins and Other Disease Associations

Pirofsky's review of early associations between diseases, cold agglutinins and hemolytic anemia included cirrhosis, pernicious anemia and various forms of carcinoma.[82] More recent work has focused on anti I^T. Garratty et al[85] were the first to draw attention to the occurrence of antibodies with I^T specificity in the serum of patients with Hodgkin's disease. The first report described anti-I^T that was optimally active at 37 C, but did not behave as an autoantibody. The patient was a Caucasian with Hodgkin's disease. A larger study by Garratty's group confirmed an association between anti-I^T and Hodgkin's disease and implicated anti-I^T in acquired hemolytic anemia.[12] Anti-I^T was found as an IgG autoantibody in each of three cases of Hodgkin's disease complicated by hemolytic anemia. Anti-I^T was not found in a fourth case with hemolytic anemia. Apparently not all cases of hemolytic anemia in Hodgkin's disease can be attributed to anti-I^T. No further examples of autoanti-I^T were found in 50 other cases of Hodgkin's disease without hemolytic anemia.

Subsequent reports of anti-I^T include the case described in 1977 by Freedman et al[86] in which autoimmune hemolytic anemia was associated with anti-I^T. The antibody was remarkable in that it was optimally reactive at 37 C, although composed of IgM. This patient did not have Hodgkin's disease. Levine and coworkers[87] have reported seven cases of Hodgkin's disease associated with a positive direct antiglobulin test. Three of the patients had overt hemolytic anemia. Red cell eluates from two of the patients with hemolytic anemia and one other contained IgG anti-I^T. Hafleigh et al[88] reported examples of IgG autoanti-I^T in three patients, none of whom had Hodgkin's disease or evidence of hemolytic anemia. These autoanti-I^T were not clinically significant as evidenced by cell survival studies. Recently, Postoway et al[89] have reported a case of hemolytic anemia associated with an IgM anti-I^T cold agglutinin that exhibited activity at 37 C. This patient had non-Hodgkin's lymphoma. Ramos and coworkers[90] described a case of fatal cold antibody autoimmune hemolytic anemia associated with anti-P and a wide thermal range cold agglutinin with serologic reactions consistent with I^T specificity. The collected case reports above suggest that I^T may be an important target of autoimmunity.

Rubin and Solomon[91] were impressed by the relationship of the high incidence of cold agglutinins in Melanesians with both malaria and hyperglobulinemia. The frequent finding of anti-i in patients with infectious mononucleosis, another condition characterized by hyperglobulinemia, prompted them to explore the incidence of anti-i in patients with alcoholic cirrhosis. Forty-seven patients were studied. Titration endpoints with cord cells were higher than with adult cells in 10 cases (21%), although no correlation between the levels of serum gammaglobulins and anti-i was seen. These authors noted that the production of cold agglutinins might be a nonspecific effect of intense synthetic activity of the reticuloendothelial system.

Ii Antigens and Disease

Several reports have established a relationship between dyserythropoiesis and disturbed synthesis of the Ii red cell determinants. Usually, this has been manifested as increased agglutinability with anti-i, which has been interpreted as reflecting an increased number of i antigen sites. Occasionally, increased agglutinability with anti-I has been recorded. Lewis, Dacie and Tills[92] tested red cell samples from a large series of patients, suffering from a variety of blood diseases, for evidence of increased agglutinability with a potent anti-I serum. The results were compared with controls from patients not suffering from blood diseases as well as controls from normal subjects and newborn infants. The red cell samples from the blood-disease patient group demonstrated enhanced agglutinability that was not confined to any one type of disorder. The authors proposed that their observations might be attributed to a minor defect of the red cell membrane or, more likely, to changes in surface structure occurring in a variety of blood diseases.

In 1964, Giblett and Crookston[93] reported results of a study of 17 patients with thalassemia major. In every case an increase in i antigen activity was observed. Titration scores with anti-I, however, were normal. Similar findings have been made in some (but not all) patients with hypoplastic anemia, sideroblastic anemia, megaloblastic anemia, chronic hemolytic anemia and acute leukemia. Cooper et al[94] demonstrated increased I and i expression using the red cells of 13 of 15 patients with sideroblastic anemia and of 7 of 8 patients with megaloblastic anemia, but not in any of 8 patients suffering from iron deficiency anemia. There was no general correlation between the degree of anemia and increased agglutinability by anti-i.

Enhanced expression of i antigen was thought to be due to membrane immaturity arising from rapid marrow transit time of the red cell. Hillman and Giblett[95] made this proposal to account for the appearance of i antigen on the red cells of a patient with hemochromatosis. The patient's marrow had been stressed by serial phlebotomies, which were performed to reduce iron stores, but which also resulted in anemia. Increased i activity was associated with red cells newly launched from the marrow. This was not the explanation offered by Cooper et al,[94] who preferred the notion that increased I and i antigenic expression was a function of disordered erythropoiesis.

Maniatis et al[96] studied the agglutinability of red cells from normal adults and patients with sickle cell anemia and sickle cell trait. The red cells of patients with sickle cell anemia (SS homozygotes) were shown to have significantly increased levels of both I and i activity; cells from heterozygotes (AS) demonstrated some increase when compared to the normal controls. No evidence to support a relationship of i antigen expression and HbF content was found. This observation was consistent with expectations based on previous experience.

Reduced (rather than increased) antigenic expression has been reported by some authors. McGinniss et al[97] observed depression of I antigenic expression in 22 of 73 patients with leukemia. Some of these patients regained I antigenic expression during remission. McGinniss and colleagues did not comment on any disturbance of ABH antigens but, in view of the biochemical relationship of ABH to Ii, it would not be surprising to observe a reciprocal loss of ABH antigenic expression. Jenkins et al[98] also reported depression of I antigen activity in a leukemic patient. In this case there was associated weakened A antigen expression. Stronger than expected i activity convinced Jenkins et al that the expected Ii relationship was maintained. I antigenic depression, however, could not be confirmed by Ducos et al[99] in a study of 56 patients with leukemia.

It has been proposed that disordered erythropoiesis results in membrane alterations, which lead to increased agglutinability by anti-I and anti-i. HEMPAS (hereditary erythroblastic multinuclearity with a positive acid serum lysis test) is a condition of dyserythropoiesis associated with red cell membrane abnormalities and increased i expression. HEMPAS is inherited as an autosomal recessive character. The disease is characterized by varying degrees of anemia, with regular blood transfusions necessary in the most severe cases. Crookston[100] reported that the red cells of HEMPAS patients were much richer in i antigen than cord cells and were unusually susceptible to lysis with both anti-I and anti-i.[101] In one remarkable case cited by Crookston and Crookston,[102] a diagnosis of HEMPAS was made when a young man developed anemia due to lysis of his red cells by anti-i formed during infectious mononucleosis. Since HEMPAS heterozygotes bind twice as much anti-i as normal cells,[103] lack of anemia in obligate heterozygotes casts doubt on the role of marrow stress as the entire explanation of increased i expression in the dyserythropoietic diseases.

Close genetic linkage appears to exist in Asia between the i phenotype in adults and congenital cataracts. Seventeen of 18 Japanese with the i phenotype, from 10 different families, were found to have congenital cataracts. Forty-five other family members were tested; all were I positive, none had cataracts.[104,105] Among Chinese in Taiwan the frequency of the i phenotype among individuals with congenital cataracts is about 5%[106]; however, no such linkage was reported in six New York Caucasians with the i phenotype.[107] Yamaguchi et al[104] proposed that their findings could be explained by either close linkage between independent *Ii* and cataract genes or alternatively, by a pleiotropic effect of the gene for i. The finding of no cataracts in the six New Yorkers seems to militate against any pleiotropic effect.

I and i antigenic structures are not confined to red cells. Lalezari and Murphy[108] demonstrated agglutination of lymphocytes by anti-I and anti-i. Unlike red cells, lymphocytes retain their i antigenic expression into adult life.[109] This is true for both B and T lymphocytes. In contrast, lymphocytes from patients with chronic lymphocytic leukemia have less i antigen than normal controls.[110]

Ii Antigens and Drug-Antibody Complexes

Several reports have suggested that the binding of drug-anti-drug complexes to the red cell membrane may be facilitated through blood group antigens. Some cases have involved the Ii antigens. Duran-Suarez and colleagues[111] reported a case study of drug-induced hemolytic anemia, involving dexchlorpheniramine maleate, in which adsorption of the immune complexes was observed only on red cells carrying the I antigen. The patient's serum and the drug would together sensitize red cells to antiglobulin serum only if the red cells used were I positive. Similarly, an eluate from the patient's red cells was active with I positive cells, but not cord cells or i adult cells. A further communication from Duran-Suarez[112] reported other cases of I-dependent binding of drug-anti-drug complexes to red cells. Sera from patients with drug-induced hemolytic anemia due to rifampicin and nitrofurantoin reacted by the indirect antiglobulin test only with I-positive red cells. Cord cells and i adult cells were nonreactive.

Habibi et al[113] described a patient who acquired an antibody against thiopental. The patient developed acute intravascular hemolysis and renal failure. Immunohematologic studies demonstrated that in the presence of thiopental the patient's serum strongly agglutinated all red cells tested with the exception of i adult and cord cells. Sandvei and coworkers reported acute intravascular hemolysis in a patient receiving Fluorouracil (5-FU) injections for rectal carcinoma.[114] A 5-FU-dependent IgM antibody was detected in the serum. Although blood group specificity was not conclusively established, the antibody did not react with cord cells. Nomifensine has been incriminated in cases of drug-induced hemolytic anemia in a large number of patients. Salama et al[115] described 13 examples of antibodies to metabolites of nomifensine that reacted with normal pooled group O red cells, but not with cord cells. Furthermore, these antibodies could be inhibited by soluble I antigen.

The precise mechanisms by which drug-induced antibodies cause in vivo hemolysis are not always clear. The finding of blood-group-specific drug-dependent antibodies may help shed light on this perplexing problem by indicating specific attachment structures on the red cell membrane.

Summary

This chapter represents an attempt to review the Ii blood group complex from a blood banker's perspective. It is necessarily a restricted view of a complex system of carbohydrate structures widely distributed in tissues and secretions. These structures are important features of erythroid maturation and differentiation that might prove to be significant implications as markers of malignant change.

The emergent view of the Ii blood group collection shows a series of abundant carbohydrate epitopes common to several established blood group systems and several membrane structures. Specificity probably depends on strict molecular arrangements, especially steric orientation associated with carbohydrate branching. No doubt further clarity will be provided by finely focused monoclonal antibodies.

Nevertheless, to the blood banker the Ii blood groups are primarily nuisance autoantibodies with no clinical significance. Occasionally, however, autoantibodies with the same specificities exist in a pathologic form capable of causing in vivo hemolysis. It is not always easy to separate the benign from the malicious, especially in the middle of the night! It is at these times that cold agglutinins provide their most lively serologic challenge. Perhaps one day a clever biochemist will provide us with sources of I substances to neutralize our problems.

Acknowledgments

I gratefully acknowledge the valuable assistance given by my esteemed colleagues Mary Kowalski and Jill Hardman. The patience and industry of my secretary Patty Aulgur are nothing short of astonishing.

References

1. Wiener AS, Unger LJ, Cohen L, Feldman J. Type-specific cold auto-antibodies as a cause of acquired hemolytic anemia and hemolytic transfusion reactions: Biologic test with bovine red cells. Ann Intern Med 1956;44:221-40.
2. Marsh WL, Jenkins WJ. Anti-i: A new cold antibody. Nature 1960;188:753.
3. Lewis M, Anstee DJ, Bird GWG, et al. Blood group terminology 1990. Vox Sang 1990;58:152-69.
4. Jenkins WJ, Marsh WL, Noades J, et al. The I antigen and antibody. Vox Sang 1960;5:97-106.
5. Tippett P, Noades J, Sanger R, et al. Further studies of the I antigen and antibody. Vox Sang 1960;5:107-21.
6. Marsh WL. Anti-i: A cold antibody defining the Ii relationship in human red cells. Br J Haematol 1961;7:200-9.

7. Jenkins WJ, Koster HG, Marsh WL, Carter RL. Infectious mononucleosis: An unsuspected source of anti-i. Br J Haematol 1965;11: 480-3.
8. Race RR, Sanger R. Blood groups in man. 5th ed. Oxford: Blackwell, 1968.
9. Curtain CC, Baumgarten A, Gorman J, et al. Cold haemagglutinins: Unusual incidence in Melanesian populations. Br J Haematol 1965; 11:471-9.
10. Booth PB, Jenkins WJ, Marsh WL. Anti-I^T: A new antibody of the I blood-group system occurring in certain Melanesian sera. Br J Haematol 1966;12:341-4.
11. Booth PB. The occurrence of weak I^T red cell antigen among Melanesians. Vox Sang 1972;22:64-72.
12. Garratty G, Petz LD, Wallerstein RO, Fudenberg HH. Autoimmune hemolytic anemia in Hodgkin's disease associated with anti-I^T. Transfusion 1974;14:226-31.
13. Layrisse Z, Layrisse M. High incidence cold autoagglutinins of anti-I^T specificity in Yanomama Indians of Venezuela. Vox Sang 1968;14:369-82.
14. Layrisse Z, Layrisse M. Cold reacting auto-antibodies in Venezuelan populations. Vox Sang 1972;22:457-68.
15. Dzierzkowa-Borodej W, Seyfried H, Nichols M, et al. The recognition of water-soluble I blood group substance. Vox Sang 1970;18: 222-34.
16. Marsh WL, Nichols ME, Allen FH. Inhibition of anti-I sera by human milk. Vox Sang 1970;18:149-54.
17. Marsh WL, Nichols ME, Reid ME. The definition of two I antigen components. Vox Sang 1971;20:209-17.
18. Dzierzkowa-Borodej W, Seyfried H, Lisowska E. Serological classification of anti-I sera. Vox Sang 1975;28:110-21.
19. Gold ER. Observations on the specificity of anti-O and anti-A_1 sera. Vox Sang 1964;9:153-9.
20. Yokoyama M. Close relationship between A and I blood groups. Nature 1965;206:411.
21. Baumgarten A, Curtain CC. A high frequency of cold agglutinins of anti-IA specificity in a New Guinea highland population. Vox Sang 1970;18:21-6.
22. Salmon C, Homberg JC, Liberge G, Delarue F. Autoanticorps à spécificités multiples, anti-HI, anti-AI, anti-BI, dans certains éluats d'anémie hémolytique. Rev Franc Etud Clin Biol 1965;5:522-5.
23. Tegoli J, Harris JP, Issitt PD, Sanders CW. Anti-IB, an expected "New" antibody detecting a joint product of the *I* and *B* genes. Vox Sang 1967;13:144-57.
24. Voak D, Lodge TW, Hopkins J, Bowley CC. A study of the antibodies of the H'O'I-B complex with special reference to their occurrence and notation. Vox Sang 1968;15:353-66.

25. Drachmann O. An autoaggressive anti-BI(O) antibody. Vox Sang 1968;14:185-93.
26. Morel P, Garratty G, Willbanks E. Another example of anti-IB. Vox Sang 1975;29:231-3.
27. Rosenfield RE, Schroeder R, Ballard R, et al. Erythrocytic antigenic determinants characteristic of H, I in the presence of H [IH], or H in the absence of i [H(i)]. Vox Sang 1964;9:415-9.
28. Marcus DM, Kabat EA, Rosenfield RE. The action of enzymes from *Clostridium tertium* on the I antigenic determinant of human erythrocytes. J Exp Med 1963;118:175-94.
29. Schmidt PJ, McGinniss MH. Differences between anti-H and anti-OI red cell antibodies. Vox Sang 1965;10:109-12.
30. Giblett ER, Hillman RS, Brooks LE. Transfusion reaction during marrow suppression in a thalassemic patient with a blood group anomaly and an unusual cold agglutinin. Vox Sang 1965;10:448-59.
31. Lodge TW, Voak D. An example of inhibitable anti-HI in a group B donor. Vox Sang 1968;14:60-2.
32. Bird GWG, Wingham J. Erythrocyte autoantibody with unusual specificity. Vox Sang 1977;32:280-2.
33. Pierce SR, Kowalski MA, Hardman JT, Beck ML. Anti-Hi: More common than previously thought (abstract)? In: Book of Abstracts from the ISBT/AABB Joint Congress. Arlington, VA: American Association of Blood Banks, 1990:79.
34. Issitt PD, Tegoli J, Jackson V, et al. Anti-IP$_1$: Antibodies that show an association between the I and P blood group systems. Vox Sang 1968;14:1-8.
35. Booth PB. Anti-I^{T}P$_1$: An antibody showing a further association between the I and P blood group systems. Vox Sang 1970;19:85-90.
36. Tegoli J, Cortez M, Jensen L, Marsh WL. A new antibody, anti-ILe^{bH}, specific for a determinant formed by the combined action of the *I*, *Le*, *Se* and *H* gene products. Vox Sang 1971;21:397-404.
37. Feizi T. The blood group Ii system: A carbohydrate antigen system defined by naturally monoclonal or oligoclonal autoantibodies of man. Immunol Commun 1981;10:127-56.
38. Hakomori S. Blood group ABH and Ii antigens of human erythrocytes: Chemistry, polymorphism, and their developmental change. Semin Hematol 1981;18:39-62.
39. Anstee DJ. Blood group-active surface molecules of the human red blood cell. Vox Sang 1990;58:1-20.
40. Hakomori S, Clausen H, Levery S. A new series of blood group A and H antigens expressed in human erythrocytes and the incompatible A antigens expressed in tumors of blood group O and B individuals. Biochem Soc Trans 1987;15:593-6.
41. Roelcke D. Cold agglutination. Transfus Med Rev 1989;3:140-66.

42. Clausen H, Hakomori S. ABH and related histo-blood group antigens; immunochemical differences in carrier isotypes and their distribution. Vox Sang 1989;56:1-20.
43. Rosse WF, Sherwood JB. Cold-reacting antibodies: Differences in the reaction of anti-I antibodies with adult and cord red blood cells. Blood 1970;36:28-42.
44. Rosse WF, Lauf PK. Reaction of cold agglutinins with I antigen solubilized from human red cells. Blood 1970;36:777-84.
45. Gardas A, Košcielak J. I-active antigen of human erythrocyte membrane. Vox Sang 1974:26;227-37.
46. Shinitzky M, Soroujon M. Passive modulation of blood group antigens. Proc Natl Acad Sci USA 1979;76:4438-40.
47. Borochov H, Shinitzky M. Vertical displacement of membrane proteins mediated by changes in microviscosity. Proc Natl Acad Sci USA 1976;73:4526-30.
48. Basu MK, Flamm M, Schachter D, et al. Effects of modulating erythrocyte membrane cholesterol on Rho(D) antigen expression. Biochem Biophys Res Commun 1980;95:887-93.
49. Flamm M, Basu MK, Schachter D, et al. Role of membrane lipids in cold agglutination of human erythrocytes. Blood 1982;60:340-5.
50. Issitt PD, Jackson VA. Useful modifications and variations of technics in work on I system antibodies. Vox Sang 1968;15:152-3.
51. Dameshek W. Cold hemagglutinins in acute hemolytic reactions in association with sulfonamide medication and infections. JAMA 1943;123:77-80.
52. Wiener AS, Gordon EB, Gallop C. Studies on autoantibodies in human sera. J Immunol 1953;71:58-65.
53. Evans RS, Turner E, Bingham M. Studies with radioiodinated cold agglutinins of ten patients. Am J Med 1965;38:378-95.
54. Petz LD, Garratty G. Acquired immune hemolytic anemias. New York: Churchill Livingstone, 1980.
55. Peterson OL, Ham TH, Finland M. Cold agglutinins (autoheamagglutinins) in primary atypical pneumonia. Science 1943;97:167.
56. Horstmann DM, Tatlock H. Cold agglutinins: A diagnostic aid in certain types of primary atypical pneumonia. JAMA 1943;122:369-70.
57. Dacie JV. The haemolytic anaemias. 2nd ed. London: J and A Churchill Ltd, 1962.
58. Tanowitz HB, Robbins N, Leidich N. Hemolytic anemia: Associated with severe mycoplasma pneumoniae pneumonia. NY State J Med 1978;78:2231-2.
59. Janney FA, Lee LT, Howe C. Cold hemagglutinin cross-reactivity with *Mycoplasma pneumoniae*. Infect Immun 1978;22:29-33.
60. Costea N, Yakulis VJ, Heller P. Inhibition of cold agglutinins (anti-I) by *M. pneumoniae* antigens. Proc Soc Exp Biol (NY) 1972;139:476-9.

61. Schmidt PJ, Barile MF, McGinniss MH. Mycoplasma (pleuropneumonia-like organisms) and blood group I; associations with neoplastic disease. Nature 1965;205:371-2.
62. Feizi T. The monoclonal antibodies of cold agglutinin syndrome. Med Biol 1980;58(3):123-7.
63. Bell CA, Zwicker H, Rosenbaum DL. Paroxysmal cold hemoglobinuria (PCH) following mycoplasma infection: Anti-I specificity of the biphasic hemolysin. Transfusion 1973;13:138-41.
64. Engelfriet CP, von dem Borne AEGKr, Moes M, van Loghem JJ. Serological studies in autoimmune haemolytic anaemia. Bibl Haematol 1968;29:473.
65. Rosenfield RE, Schmidt PJ, Calvo RC, McGinniss MH. Anti-i, a frequent cold agglutinin in infectious mononucleosis. Vox Sang 1965;10:631-4.
66. Worlledge SM, Dacie JV. Haemolytic and other anaemias in infectious mononucleosis. In: Carter HG, Penman RL, eds. Infectious mononucleosis. Oxford: Blackwell Scientific, 1969.
67. Hoagland RJ. Infectious mononucleosis. New York: Grune and Stratton, 1967.
68. Horwitz CA, Moulds J, Henle W, et al. Cold agglutinins in infectious mononucleosis and heterophil-antibody-negative mononucleosis-like syndromes. Blood 1977;50:195-202.
69. Troxel DB, Innella F, Cohen RJ. Infectious mononucleosis complicated by hemolytic anemia due to anti-i. Am J Clin Pathol 1966;46:625-31.
70. Goldberg LS, Barnett EV. The role of rheumatoid (antiglobulin) factors in hemolytic anemia. Ann NY Acad Sci 1969;168:122-5.
71. Capra JD, Dowling P, Cook S, Kunkel HG. An incomplete cold reactive gamma G antibody with i specificity in infectious mononucleosis. Vox Sang 1969;16:10-17.
72. Gronemeyer P, Chaplin H, Ghazarian V, et al. Hemolytic anemia complicating infectious mononucleosis due to the interaction of an IgG cold anti-i and an IgM cold rheumatoid factor. Transfusion 1981;21:715-18.
73. Wilkinson LS, Petz LD, Garratty G. Reappraisal of the role of anti-i in haemolytic anaemia in infectious mononucleosis. Br J Haematol 1973;25:715-22.
74. Burkart PT, Hsu TCS. IgM cold-warm hemolysins in infectious mononucleosis. Transfusion 1979;19:535-8.
75. Finland M, Barnes MW. Cold agglutinins VIII. Arch Intern Med 1958;101:462-6.
76. Laroche C, Milliez P, Dreyfus B, et al. Ictère hémolytique aigu post-grippal. Bull Soc Med Hop, Paris 1951;67:779.
77. Ventura S, Aresu G. Grave anemia immuno-emolitica in decorso di influenza cosidetta "asiatica." Rass Med Sarda, 1957;59:609.

78. Puxeddu A, Colonua A, Nenci GG et al. Su di un raro caso di anemia emolitica autoimmune da virus influenzale B. Haematologica 1965;50:1073.
79. Dausset J, Colombani J. The serology and the prognosis of 128 cases of autoimmune hemolytic anemia. Blood 1959;14:1280-1301.
80. Betke K, Richarz H, Schubothe H, Vivell O. Beobachtungen zu Krankheitsbild, Pathogenese und Atiologie der akuten erworbenen hämolytischen Anämie (Lederer-anämie). Klin Wschr 1953;31:373-80.
81. Pien FD, Smith TF, Taswell HF, et al. Cold-reactive antibodies in a case of congenital cytomegalovirus infection. Am J Clin Pathol 1974;61:352-7.
82. Pirofsky B. Autoimmunization and the autoimmune hemolytic anemias. Baltimore: Williams and Wilkins Company, 1969.
83. Marienberg G. Kält-Agglutinine bei Trypanosomiasis und Malaria. Z Tropenmed Parasitol 1951;3:33-41.
84. Korn RJ, Yakulis VJ, Lemke CE, Chaomet B. Cold agglutinins in *Listeria monocytogenes* infections. Arch Intern Med 1957;99:573-80.
85. Garratty G, Hafleigh B, Dalziel J, Petz LD. An IgG anti-I^T detected in a Caucasian American. Transfusion 1972;12:325-9.
86. Freedman J, Newlands M, Johnson CA. Warm IgM anti-I^T causing autoimmune haemolytic anaemia. Vox Sang 1977;32:135-42.
87. Levine AM, Thornton P, Forman SJ, et al. Positive Coombs test in Hodgkin's disease: Significance and implications. Blood 1980;55:607-11.
88. Hafleigh EB, Wells RF, Grumet FC. Nonhemolytic IgG anti-I^T. Transfusion 1978;18:592-7.
89. Postoway N, Capon S, Smith L, et al. Cold agglutinin syndrome caused by anti-I^T (abstract). In: Book of Abstracts from the ISBT/AABB Joint Congress. Arlington, VA: American Association of Blood Banks, 1990:85.
90. Ramos RR, Curtis BR, Eby CS, et al. Fatal autoimmune hemolytic anemia (AHA) associated with IgM bi-thermic anti-P and cold I^T antibodies (abstract). In: Book of Abstracts ISBT/AABB Joint Congress. Arlington, VA: American Association of Blood Banks, 1990:86.
91. Rubin H, Solomon A. Cold agglutinins of anti-i specificity in alcoholic cirrhosis. Vox Sang 1967;12:227-30.
92. Lewis SM, Dacie JV, Tills D. Comparison of the sensitivity to agglutination and haemolysis by a high-titre cold antibody of the erythrocytes of normal subjects and of patients with a variety of blood diseases including paroxysmal nocturnal haemoglobinuria. Br J Haematol 1961;7:64-72.

93. Giblett ER, Crookson MC. Agglutinability of red cells by anti-i in patients with thalassaemia major and other haematological disorders. Nature 1964;201:1138-9.
94. Cooper AG, Hoffbrand AV, Worlledge SM. Increased agglutinability by anti-i of red cells in sideroblastic and megaloblastic anaemia. Br J Haematol 1968;15:381-7.
95. Hillman RS, Giblett ER. Red cell membrane alteration associated with "marrow stress." J Clin Invest 1965;44:1730-6.
96. Maniatis A, Frieman B, Bertles JF. Increased expression in erythrocytic Ii antigens in sickle cell disease and sickle cell trait. Vox Sang 1977;33:29-36.
97. McGinniss MH, Schmidt PJ, Carbone PP. Close association of I blood group and disease. Nature 1964;202:606.
98. Jenkins WJ, Marsh WL, Gold ER. Reciprocal relationship of antigens "I" and "i" in health and disease. Nature 1965;205:813.
99. Ducos J, Ruffie J, Colombies P, et al. I antigen in leukaemic patients. Nature 1965;208:1329-30.
100. Crookston JH, Crookston MC, Burnie KL, et al. Hereditary erythroblastic multinuclearity associated with a positive acidified-serum test: A type of congenital dyserythropoietic anaemia. Br J Haematol 1969;17:11-26.
101. Crookston JH, Godwin TF, Wightman KJR, et al. Congenital dyserythropoietic anaemia (abstract). Eleventh Congress, Sydney. International Society of Haematology, 1966:18.
102. Crookston JH, Crookston MC. HEMPAS: Clinical, hematological and serological features. In: Charles Salmon, ed. Blood groups and other red cell surface markers in health and disease. New York: Masson, 1982:29-38.
103. Crookston JH, Crookston MC, Rosse WF. Red cell membrane abnormalities in hereditary erythroblastic multinuclearity (abstract). Blood 1969;34:844.
104. Yamaguchi H, Okubo Y, Tomita M. A note on possible close linkage between the Ii blood locus and a congenital cataract locus. Proc Japan Acad 1979;48:625-8.
105. Ogata H, Okubo Y, Akabane T. Phenotype i associated with congenital cataract in Japanese. Transfusion 1979;19:166-8.
106. Lin-Chu M, Broadberry RE, Tanaka M, Okubo Y. The rare ii phenotype and congenital cataract among Chinese in Taiwan (abstract). In: Book of Abstracts from the ISBT/AABB Joint Congress. Arlington, VA: American Association of Blood Banks, 1990:155.
107. Marsh WL, DePalma H. Association between the Ii blood group and congenital cataract. Transfusion 1982;22:337-8.
108. Lalezari P, Murphy GB. Cold reacting leukocyte agglutinins and their significance. In: Curtoni ES, Mattiuz PL, Tosi RM. Histocompatibility testing. Copenhagen: Munksgaard, 1967:421.

109. Shumak KH, Rachkewich RA, Crookston MC, Crookston JH. Antigens of the Ii system on lymphocytes. Nature (New Biol) 1971;231: 148-9.
110. Pruzanski W, Shumak KH. Biologic activity of cold-reacting autoantibodies. N Engl J Med 1977;297:583-9.
111. Duran-Suarez JR, Martin-Vega C, Argelagues E, et al. The I antigen as an immune complex receptor in a case of haemolytic anaemia induced by an antihistaminic agent. Br J Haematol 1981;49:153-4.
112. Duran-Suarez JR, Martin-Vega C, Argelagues E, et al. Red cell I antigen as immune complex receptor in drug-induced hemolytic anemias. Vox Sang 1981;41:313-5.
113. Habibi B, Basty R, Chodez S, Prunat A. Thiopental-related immune hemolytic anemia and renal failure. Specific involvement of red cell antigen I. N Engl J Med 1985;312:353-5.
114. Sandvei P, Nordhagen R, Michaelsen TE, Wolthuis K. Fluorouracil (5-FU) induced acute immune haemolytic anaemia. Br J Haematol 1987;65:357-9.
115. Salama A, Mueller-Eckhardt C. On the mechanisms of sensitization and attachment of antibodies to RBC in drug-induced immune hemolytic anemia. Blood 1987;69:1006-10.

In: Moulds JM and Woods LL, eds.
Blood Groups: P, I, Sd^a and Pr
Arlington, VA: American Association of Blood Banks, 1991

3

The Antigens Sd^a and Cad

Peter D. Issitt, PhD, FIMLS, FIBiol, CBiol, FRCPath

IN 1967, IN BACK TO BACK papers, Macvie et al[1] and Renton et al[2] described a new antibody, anti-Sd^a. It was suggested that if the system to which Sd^a belonged was found to be independent of others it be called Sid. While Sd^a remains genetically independent of all known blood group systems, the International Society of Blood Transfusion (ISBT) Working Party on Terminology for Red Cell Surface Antigens has categorized it as a high-incidence antigen not assigned to a system or a collection. The number 901012 has been assigned to the antigen.[3] From the early studies,[1,2] it appeared that Sd^a had an incidence of about 91% in the predominantly White English population studied. However, as described in more detail below, it was later found[4] that among individuals whose red cells type as Sd(a–), a little over half secrete Sd^a substance in the urine, and in smaller amounts in the saliva. Thus, the true incidence of the Sd(a+) phenotype is around 96%. As far as this author has been able to determine, no significant differences from that incidence have been found in other populations. Again, as discussed in more detail later, a small proportion of persons with Sd(a+) red cells (around 1% in the initial studies) have an exceptionally strong expression of the antigen on their cells. This phenotype is often written as Sd(a++) and in everyday parlance is called "super Sid."[5] At one time it was believed[6] that the Sd(a++) and Cad+ phenotypes (see below) were the same thing. Thus, "super Sid" appeared to be more common in Thailand than elsewhere.[7,8] However, it is no longer certain that Sd^a and Cad are the same. The fact that the two share a common immunodominant structure may explain their close similarity at the serologic level. While all individuals have a serum antibody that agglutinates Cad-polyagglutinable red cells it seems that anti-Sd^a, as demonstrable by conventional serologic techniques, is made only by persons with Sd(a–) red cells whose saliva and urine lack Sd^a substance.

Peter D. Issitt, PhD, FIMLS, FIBiol, CBiol, FRCPath, Associate Professor of Pathology and Scientific Director, Immunohematology, Transfusion Service, Duke University Medical Center, Durham, North Carolina

Sd^a

The Sd^a Antigen

On Human Red Blood Cells

From the time that it was first reported, it was apparent that the Sd^a antigen is unusual in a number of respects. First, even when red cells with a well-developed form of the antigen are tested, they give a mixed-field reaction with anti-Sd^a. The typical picture is a number of tight agglutinates superimposed on a field of unagglutinated red cells. However, if the agglutinates are removed and the previously unagglutinated red cells are exposed to the same anti-Sd^a, additional agglutinates are formed. Thus, it seems that all the red cells of a person with the Sd(a+) phenotype carry the antigen; it has been suggested[2] that distribution of the antigen varies among the red cells. Such distribution is not related to red cell age; when young and older red cells are separated by centrifugation, both populations show the mixed-field reaction.[2,5]

Second, there is great variation in strength of the Sd^a antigen on the red cells of different individuals. As mentioned, about 1% of persons have red cells that are so strongly agglutinated (albeit still with a mixed-field pattern) that they are called Sd(a++). In 80% of persons the antigen can be shown to be present but the positive reactions are weaker. In 10% of persons the antigen is detected with difficulty due to very weak reactions. In the next 5% of persons the red cells type as Sd(a–), even when potent anti-Sd^a is used, but Sd^a substance can be found in the urine. Because inhibition studies using urine have shown such individuals to be phenotypically Sd(a+), no attempts to adsorb and/or elute anti-Sd^a with such cells seem to have been reported. This leaves, of course, about 4% of persons who are truly Sd(a–) since their red cells, urine and saliva all lack the antigen. The findings described are summarized in Table 3-1. Although it is convenient to divide persons as shown in the table, distribution of Sd^a on the red cells of different individuals actually represents a sliding scale from 4+ to negative.

Third, although some 96% of persons are genetically Sd(a+) there is a marked loss of antigen expression during pregnancy. In different studies, 75%,[9] 48%[1] and 36%[10] of women at full term were found to have red cells that typed as Sd(a–). The differences may have been due in part to the abilities of different anti-Sd^a to react with red cells carrying low levels of the antigen. In their study, Morton and Pickles[9] found that the Sd(a–) phenotype persisted for at least 6 weeks after delivery in 25% of women. Spitalnik et al[10] found that in the first trimester of pregnancy, 22 of 100 women had the Sd(a–) phenotype. Of 145 women tested at full term, 52 (36%) were Sd(a–). Thus, loss of Sd^a antigen expression seems to be progressive as pregnancy advances. In spite of the marked increase of the Sd(a–) phenotype in pregnancy, the incidence of anti-Sd^a was no different

Table 3-1. Sd^a Phenotypes

Reaction of RBCs With Anti-Sd^a	Sd^a in Saliva and Urine	Phenotype	Percent of Population
4+	Yes	Sd(a++)	1
1+ to 3+*	Yes	Sd(a+)	80
±†	Yes	Sd(a+)	10
0	Yes	Sd(a+)	5
0‡	No	Sd(a−)	4

*In the 80% of persons whose red cells give 1＋ to 3＋ reactions with anti-Sd^a, more give 1+ than give 3+ reactions.

†In the 10% of persons whose red cells give ± reactions with anti-Sd^a, presence of the antigen on red cells may be demonstrable only with potent anti-Sd^a.

‡Anti-Sd^a in a form demonstrable in conventional serologic techniques is made only by persons who lack Sd^a from their red cells, saliva and urine.

among pregnant and nonpregnant persons studied.[10] As discussed above and mentioned in Table 3-1, it seems that only those persons who are genetically Sd(a−) and whose saliva and urine lack Sd^a form the antibody. Loss of Sd^a from the red cells during pregnancy is not accompanied by loss of Sd^a substance from the saliva and urine.

Fourth, the Sd^a antigen is not developed on the red cells of newborn infants. Cord blood samples invariably type as Sd(a−); in infants who have inherited an Sd^a gene, red cell expression of the antigen is not usually readily detectable until about 10 weeks of age.[9] This finding contrasts sharply with the presence of large amounts of Sd^a in the saliva of newborns (see below).

Sources of Soluble Sd^a

As mentioned above, Morton and Pickles[4] showed that Sd^a is widely distributed in the secretions, excretions and tissues of Sd(a+) persons. The largest amounts were found in urine but saliva, meconium and milk all contained enough Sd^a substance to effect some inhibition of anti-Sd^a. Serum from Sd(a+) persons was also found to contain Sd^a substance[4]; much larger quantities were found in the sera of Sd(a++) persons.[5] In using extracts from various tissues, evidence for the presence of Sd^a in the kidney, stomach, colon and lymph nodes was obtained; extracts made from the duodenum, jejunum, ileum, liver, spleen, muscles and brain were not inhibitory. In other species, Sd^a substance was found in the kidneys of guinea pigs, moles and hedgehogs but not in that of a lamb. Sd^a was not found in birds; chickens, turkeys, pheasants, wood pigeons and a tawny owl were tested.

These findings have led to a number of applications at the practical level. First, the most reliable way to determine an individual's phenotype when red cell typings give equivocal (or negative) results is to use the individual's urine in a hemagglutination inhibition study of anti-Sd^a. Second, when an antibody is suspected of having anti-Sd^a specificity but the point has not been completely proved, inhibition studies using human or guinea pig urine can be used. Of the various secretions and tissue extracts listed above, guinea pig urine was shown[4] to contain the highest level of Sd^a substance. Details of methods used to perform Sd^a typing by urine inhibition, the use of guinea pig urine to confirm the specificity of anti-Sd^a and the preparation of urine samples so that they do not cause nonspecific inhibition, are given in Chapter 5. Third, the finding that Sd^a was not present in the chicken explained an earlier observation[5] that a chicken, immunized with human red cells, made anti-Sd^a.

As described above, there is a marked loss of red cell Sd^a antigen expression in pregnancy and the red cells of newborn infants type as Sd(a−). Both observations relate to red cell antigen expression only. The urine of pregnant women and newborns continues to contain Sd^a substance and the level of Sd^a in the saliva of infants is about four times greater than that in the saliva of adults.[4] Loss of red cell Sd^a antigen in pregnancy is reminiscent of the loss of red cell Le^b and reduced production of *A* gene-specified transferase in the same situation. Indeed, as detailed in the section on biochemistry of the Sd^a and Cad antigens, the Sd^a immunodominant sugar is added by an N-acetylgalactosaminyltransferase. While Howell[11] showed that the level of Sd^a in an individual's plasma is directly proportional to the amount on the individual's red cells, incubation of Sd(a−) red cells in plasma from Sd(a+) and Sd(a++) persons did not result in the cells acquiring Sd^a.[1,5] Possible explanations for this difference from the Lewis system are discussed in the section on biochemistry.

Anti-Sd^a

Detection

There is no doubt that most examples of anti-Sd^a are of the non-red-cell-stimulated (ie, naturally occurring) type. Of the 4% of persons who have Sd(a−) red cells and no Sd^a in the urine, about one quarter[2] to one half[4] have anti-Sd^a in the serum. That is to say, the antibody can be found in 1-2% of random individuals. However, the antibody is detected with this frequency only when Sd(a++) red cells are used for antibody screening. If Sd(a+) red cells of moderate antigen strength are used in such tests, most examples of the antibody go unnoticed. Virtually all the early[1,2,9] reported examples of anti-Sd^a (and many described since) were IgM in nature. Most of them presented as agglutinins, optimally reactive at around 20 C, although they were also detectable in indirect antiglobulin tests (IATs) if anti-IgM was present in the antiglobulin reagent or if anti-C3 was present and the anti-Sd^a were tested in a system that allowed them to activate complement.[9] The antibody reacts with enzyme-treated red cells and rare examples, when fresh, may cause in vitro hemolysis of such cells.[9,12] As far as this author has been able to determine, treatment of red cells with 2-aminoethylisothiouronium bromide (AET) does not denature the Sd^a antigen. One of the more useful clues in the identification of anti-Sd^a is that it is one of relatively few antibodies to common antigens that react by IATs that fails to react with cord blood red cells.

Another factor that contributes to the paucity of examples of anti-Sd^a now detected is that currently used serologic methods are not particularly favorable for its detection. The antibody usually reacts optimally at temperatures below 37 C. Even when it is detected in IATs, it is often found because the cell-serum mixtures converted to IATs were previously incubated, or left to stand, at room temperature. In methods such as low ionic strength saline (LISS), polyethylene glycol (PEG) and Polybrene® in which short (or no) incubation below 37 C is used, too little anti-Sd^a may bind for subsequent detection. Further, many workers read such tests with anti-IgG so that anti-Sd^a will not be detected via the C3-anti-C3 reaction. Failure to detect such examples of anti-Sd^a is clearly an advantage. As discussed in detail below, anti-Sd^a is almost always a clinically benign antibody. As with any antibody of that type, nondetection is an advantage since the work involved in antibody identification and possible delays in transfusion while the antibody is being identified are avoided.

As with most examples of cold-reactive, clinically insignificant antibodies, the strength and immunoglobulin class of most examples of anti-Sd^a do not change in persons transfused with Sd(a+) blood. Although some exceptions are described below, even those have not been associated with immediate or delayed hemolytic transfusion reactions. In 1978, Silvergleid et al[13] described three examples of anti-Sd^a that included IgM and IgG components and one that was solely IgG. In 1982, Spitalnik et al[10] studied the sera of six patients with anti-Sd^a who had received Sd(a+) blood. In three of them no change in the strength of the antibody was associated with the transfusion. In the other three the antibody titers did increase and much of the increase represented IgG anti-Sd^a. However, in neither of these studies was there any evidence that the anti-Sd^a had destroyed antigen-positive red cells in vivo.

Lack of Clinical Significance

As will be apparent from what has been written in the preceding section, anti-Sd^a is usually of no clinical significance. That is to say, it is usually incapable of bringing about accelerated in vivo clearance of Sd(a+) red cells. In the first two reports about the antibody, the authors[1,2] commented that since the antibody is relatively common and since 96% of random donors have the Sd(a+) phenotype, many persons with anti-Sd^a in the serum must have been transfused with Sd(a+) blood, even before those reports appeared. As with the patients studied in those two investigations, none had been described as having any untoward reaction. Further, although anti-Sd^a was identified in the sera of many pregnant women, no example caused hemolytic disease of the newborn.

In the patients studied by Silvergleid et al,[13] in vivo red cell survival studies using ^{51}Cr-labeled Sd(a+) red cells were performed. Although all four patients had at least some IgG anti-Sd^a, the 1-hour survival rate of the injected red cells was normal in each case. Three of the patients were subsequently transfused with a total of 13 Sd(a+) units between them. In all three the expected posttransfusion hematocrit levels were seen. In the fourth patient, who had IgM and IgG anti-Sd^a, the ^{51}Cr-labeled red cell survival study was done with Sd(a++) red cells. One hour following the injection, 92% of the injected red cells were still present in the patient's circulation.

Somewhat similarly, although they did not perform in vivo red cell survival studies with labeled red cells, Spitalnik et al[10] reported that in their six patients with anti-Sd^a who were transfused with Sd(a+) blood, the expected rises in posttransfusion hematocrit were seen and that neither clinical nor laboratory evidence of immune-mediated red cell destruction was found.

In 1973, College et al[14] described a case in which a patient with anti-Sd^a was transfused with 14 units of Sd(a+) blood during open-heart surgery. Red cell survival studies and careful posttransfusion evaluation indicated normal survival of the transfused red cells. In this case, the patient's IgM anti-Sd^a showed no change in immunoglobulin class or strength after the transfusions.

There must, by now, be hundreds of cases similar to those described above in which patients with anti-Sd^a have been transfused with Sd(a+) blood with an entirely satisfactory outcome. This author has personal experience of several and has heard anecdotal reports of many others. Because the benign nature of anti-Sd^a is so clearly established, such cases no longer need to be reported in the literature.

The one report in the literature of a transfusion reaction caused by anti-Sd^a is that of Peetermans and Cole-Dergent.[15] The patient involved was given seven units of blood with no untoward reactions. Ten days later he was transfused again because of renewed gastric hemorrhage. This time he had an urticarial reaction to the first unit given and a hemolytic reaction to the fourth. His serum was found to contain an IgM anti-Sd^a; all blood given was shown to have been Sd(a+). A ^{51}Cr-labeled red cell survival study, using Sd(a+) red cells that were not of the Sd(a++) phenotype, showed a two-component curve. Fifty percent of the small dose of injected cells was cleared with T1/2 of 2 days; the remaining cells survived normally (T1/2, 27 days). It was then shown that the donor's red cells that caused the reaction were of the Sd(a++) phenotype. The lesson from this case seems clear. Once identified, anti-Sd^a can be ignored for transfusion purposes providing that compatibility tests show only average reactivity indicating that the units to be used are of the Sd(a+) phenotype. In the rare event that a unit tested with the patient's serum shows strong reactivity, and may thus be of the Sd(a++) phenotype, that unit should not be given. This means that in patients with identified anti-Sd^a, only about one unit in 100 need be regarded as incompatible. For patients in whom anti-Sd^a has not been detected and who will receive blood tested for compatibility only by an immediate-spin method, the danger of a transfusion reaction must be virtually nonexistent because of weakness of the antibody and its restricted thermal range.

Some Other Findings About Sd^a

In one of the initial studies[1] on Sd^a, it was noted that saliva samples from group A persons seemed to contain more Sd^a than those from persons of other ABO groups. Although secretors of ABH substances tended to have more Sd^a substance in the saliva than did nonsecretors, there was no correlation between the levels of A, B or H and Sd^a. Similarly, the level of Sd^a secreted was not correlated with the level of Le^b in saliva. In both initial studies[1,2] it was reported that Sd^a was genetically independent of the ABO system (and of many others) and that there was no disturbance in the incidence of the Sd(a+) and Sd(a−) phenotypes based on ABO groups. In retrospect, it seems likely that the early hints of some similarity between Sd^a and A were related to the biochemical structures of the antigens.

In 1973, Lewis et al[16] described a family in which "super Sid" and Wr^a were segregating. The count of six nonrecombinants to no recombinants was just short of statistical significance. As far as this author has been able to determine, no further information about this fascinating hint of linkage has become available.

As mentioned briefly above, information about the biochemical structure of the Sd^a antigen is now available. Because of close similarities between Sd^a and another red cell antigen, Cad, some serologic information about Cad will be presented before the biochemical findings are considered.

Cad

The Antigen Cad

In 1968, Cazal et al[17] described the first example of polyagglutination of an inherited variety. The polyagglutinable red cells were said to carry the low-incidence antigen Cad that was inherited as a Mendelian dominant character, and it was concluded that all normal sera contain some anti-Cad. Since that time, graded expressions of the Cad antigen on red cells that are not polyagglutinable have been found, leading to designations of the phenotypes Cad 1, 2, 3 and 4.[18,19] In the phenotypes Cad 1 (polyagglutinable) and Cad 2 (not polyagglutinable) the Cad antigen can be recognized on group O and group B samples because the red cells are agglutinated by *Dolichos biflorus* at a dilution at which that lectin is normally used as anti-A_1. In the phenotypes Cad 3 and Cad 4, the red cells are agglutinated by potent anti-Cad but not by *D. biflorus*. In 1971, Sanger et al[6] showed that Cad 1 red cells behave as Sd(a++) and that Sd(a++) red cells are agglutinated by the *D. biflorus* lectin. It was concluded that Cad and Sd^a are the same antigen and that the Cad antigen, at its highest level "is Sd^a in excelsis."[5] This meant, of course, since Cad 1 red cells are polyagglutinable, that all sera from Sd(a+) persons must contain some anti-Sd^a. Race and Sanger[5] likened the situation to the presence of anti-A_1 in persons who are group A_2 or A_2B or the situation in which careful tests detect anti-H in most sera.[20] Since there is now some doubt as to whether the normal incomplete "cold" anti-H is truly an antibody,[12] this author preferred[21] to liken the presence of some anti-Sd^a in the sera of all Sd(a+) persons to the presence of low levels of (clinically benign) anti-I in all persons with I+ red cells.[22] The question now seems somewhat moot. Although there are marked similarities between Sd^a and Cad and while it is still possible that the two are the same thing, linkage of the antigen-bearing structures to N-glycans and O-glycans respectively[23] suggests that the transferase enzymes that add the immunodominant sugar may have slightly different specificities.

Because this chapter deals primarily with Sd^a and since Cad is included only because of its serologic and biochemical similarity to Sd(a++) full details about the Cad 1 to 4 phenotypes will not be given. However, Table 3-2 shows the reactions of some lectins with Cad+ and Sd(a++) red cells. The table is excerpted from a larger one, published elsewhere.[21] Readers requiring more information about lectin specificities and the Cad phenotypes are referred to that publication. As the later section on biochemistry in this chapter will make clear, the positive reactions listed in Table 3-2 represent the fact that Sd^a and Cad both have N-acetylgalactosamine as their immunodominant character.

Table 3-2. The Reactions of Group A Red Cells and Group O or B Red Cells That Are Sd(a++) or Carry Cad or Tn, With Selected Sera and Lectins

Reagent	Red Cell Phenotype			
	A	Sd(a++)	Cad+[§]	Tn+[‖]
Human serum from non-immunized group A and AB individuals	0	0	+	+[¶]
Human anti-Sd^a*	0–2+	4+	4+	+
Dolichos biflorus†	+	+	+	+
Salvia sclarea	0	0	0	+
Salvia horminum‡	0	+	+	+

*Reactions of human anti-Sd^a will vary based on strength of the antibody and the expression of Sd^a on the group A and Tn+ red cells.
†Dolichos biflorus lectin can be diluted to a point at which it will agglutinate A$_1$ but not A$_2$ red cells. At that dilution it will still agglutinate Sd(a++), most Cad 1 and 2 and Tn+ red cells.
‡Salvia horminum is said to contain separable anti-Cad and anti-Tn. Presumably, it is the anti-Cad component that agglutinates Sd(a++) red cells.
§In this table the Cad+ phenotype indicates Cad-polyagglutinable red cells.
‖Tn+ red cells are also polyagglutinable.
¶Reactions shown as + will vary from 1+ to 4+ dependent on the reagents used.

Biochemistry

Sd^a

The finding[4] that urine from individuals with Sd(a+) red cells contains large amounts of a substance capable of specific inhibition of anti-Sd^a provided biochemists with starting material for studies designed to elucidate the structure of the Sd^a antigen. As early as 1970, Morton and Terry[24] achieved partial purification of the Sd^a-bearing material and showed that it could be separated from A substance in urine. The observation was important since both Sd^a and A have N-acetylgalactosamine (GalNAc) as a terminal nonreducing carbohydrate. Between 1979 and 1981, Morgan et al[25,26] and Soh et al[27] provided evidence that the Tamm and Horsfall (T-H) urinary glycoprotein is the major carrier of Sd^a in the urine. The T-H glycoprotein had, of course, been recognized and partially characterized many years earlier.[28,29] Soh et al[27] showed that in the urine of persons with Sd(a+) red cells, the T-H glycoprotein contains some 1-2% of GalNAc. In the urine of persons with Sd(a–) red cells, the GalNAc content is less than 0.2%. Antibody inhibition[5,6] and lectin (see Table 3-2) studies had, of course, already provided indirect evidence of a role for GalNAc, probably as one of the immunodominant carbohydrates, in Sd^a structure. However, as blood group serologists are well aware, GalNAc is immunodominant in (at least) A, Tn, P and the Forssman antigens, yet antibodies to those antigens differ from each other and from anti-Sd^a. GalNAc is also immunodominant in the Cad antigen but it is much harder to decide if anti-Sd^a and anti-Cad are different from each other. The combined serologic and biochemical studies thus showed that Sd^a is not simply GalNAc as a terminal residue on the T-H urinary glycoprotein.

Donald et al[30] isolated the disaccharide GalNAcβ(1→4)Gal from the T-H glycoprotein in the urine of persons with Sd(a+) red cells. It was found that this disaccharide inhibited *D. biflorus* lectin but not human anti-Sd^a. This reflects the fact that lectins invariably have a more simple specificity than do human antibodies. *D. biflorus* is known[31] to complex with both N-acetyl-α and β-D-galactosamine. Clearly anti-Sd^a requires more than just terminal GalNAc in the structure to which it binds. Donald et al[32] then isolated the pentasaccharide GalNAcβ(1→4)[Neu-Acα(2→3)]-Galβ(1→4)GlcNAcβ(1→3)Gal from the same source as they had used to isolate the disaccharide. This pentasaccharide was shown to inhibit both *D. biflorus* and human anti-Sd^a.

Next, Williams et al,[33] in a nuclear magnetic resonance study of oligosaccharides isolated from the T-H glycoprotein in the urine of persons with Sd(a+) red cells, showed that the pentasaccharide listed above includes the branched terminal trisaccharide GalNAcβ(1→4)[Neu-Acα(2→3)]Gal. This trisaccharide also inhibits anti-Sd^a; further, the inhibitory ability is lost if either the GalNAc or the NeuAc (sialic acid) residue is removed.[30,34,35]

The pentasaccharide mentioned above and the trisaccharide contained therein that is capable of inhibiting anti-Sd^a are depicted in Fig 3-1. To a simple-minded serologist, such as this author, the findings described seem to show that while the terminal GalNAc in Fig 3-1 is the immunodominant structure in the Sd^a antigen in urine, both the NeuAc and the subterminal Gal are required for complete expression of Sd^a. As with antigens of other systems that require more than one carbohydrate for full integrity, this seems to suggest either that the additional carbohydrates are necessary for antibody binding to occur (ie, they are part of the antigen) or that their presence is essential for the terminal carbohydrate (in this case GalNAc) to be presented in the correct spatial orientation for antibody recognition to occur.

Naturally, since the immunodominant sugar of Sd^a was shown to be GalNAc, efforts were made to isolate and characterize the transferase enzyme responsible for addition of the terminal GalNAc residue. Three groups of workers[36-38] isolated the transferase. Donald et al[37] showed it to

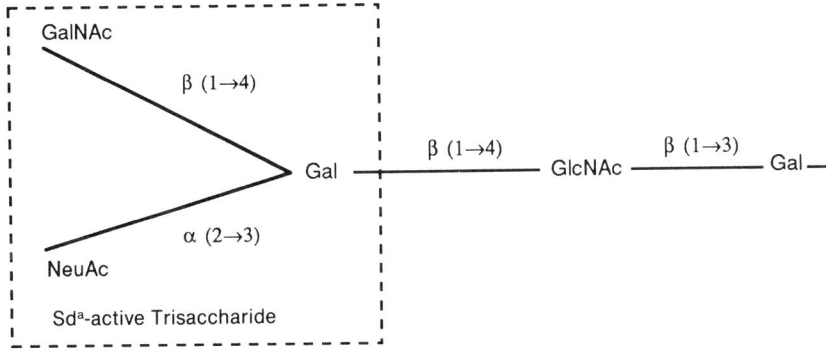

Figure 3-1. The structure of the Sd^a-containing pentasaccharide present in the T-H urinary glycoprotein. In other structures on the T-H glycoprotein the GlcNAc residue is in α(1→2) or α(1→4) linkage to mannose. GalNAc = N-acetyl-D-galactosamine, NeuAc = N-acetylneuraminic acid, Gal = D-galactose, GlcNAc = N-acetyl-D-glucosamine.

be present in urine of persons with Sd(a+) red cells but missing from urine of those whose cells are Sd(a−), while Serafini-Cessi and Dall'Olio[36] found it in the kidneys of guinea pigs. More recently, Serafini-Cessi et al[39] have further characterized the transferase and their findings with some others provide a basis for the possibility that Sd^a and Cad are different.

The finding that Sd^a antigen structure is in large part dependent on the addition of terminal GalNAc by a transferase enzyme also throws light on the finding that there is a dramatic loss of red cell Sd^a antigen expression during pregnancy. It has been shown[40,41] that in pregnancy there is a marked reduction of production of the A gene-specified enzyme, which is also an N-acetylgalactosaminyltransferase. In contrast, loss of Lewis system antigen expression in pregnancy seems to occur because an increase in plasma lipoproteins results in repartition of the Lewis-antigen-bearing structures between the red cells and plasma.[42] The situation involving loss of red cell expression of Sd^a during pregnancy seems more closely to parallel reduction of production of a transferase than competition for available antigen. Such an assumption is further supported by the finding[1,5] that Sd(a−) red cells incubated in plasma that contains Sd^a substance do not become Sd(a+). Conversion of Le(b−) red cells to the Le(b+) phenotype by incubation of those cells in plasma that contains Le^b substance represents incorporation of Le^b-bearing glycolipids by the red cells.[42] In contrast, it seems that the Sd(a+) phenotype must always be transferase-driven and that, unlike Le^b, Sd^a cannot be passively acquired by red cells.

Before leaving the subject of urinary Sd^a, it should be added that the T-H glycoprotein is not the only site at which the antigen is found in the urine. Cartron and Blanchard[43] showed that a mucin-type glycoprotein that is present in trace amounts in urine also carries Sd^a.

Cad

Unlike the situation with Sd^a, biochemical characterization of the Cad antigen was accomplished using red cell membranes as the starting material. Serologic studies[6,44,45] strongly suggested that as in Sd^a (and at least the A, Tn, P and Forssman antigens) the immunodominant carbohydrate in Cad is GalNAc. Cartron and Blanchard[43] found that in sodium dodecylsulfate polyacrylamide gel electrophoresis (SDS-PAGE) studies, both glycophorins A and B (the MN and Ss sialoglycoproteins, for a review see reference 21) from Cad+ red cells had decreased mobility, as compared to those from Cad– cells, suggesting an increased molecular mass of the glycophorins on Cad+ cells. Analysis of purified glycophorin A from Cad+ red cells revealed an increase in GalNAc content and normal NeuAc content as compared to Cad– cells. Since it was already well-established (again see reference 21 for a review and references) that glycophorin A carries up to 15 copies of a tetrasaccharide side chain that normally includes only one GalNAc residue, the equivalent side chains isolated from glycophorin A from Cad+ red cells were analyzed. Blanchard et al[46] found that in many of the side chains a second GalNAc residue was present in β(1→4) linkage to Gal. Figure 3-2 illustrates the usual tetrasaccharide found on glycophorins A and B of Cad– red cells, the pentasaccharide found on Cad+ cells and the disaccharide found on Tn cells. Herkt et al[47] isolated and separated the oligosaccharide side chains of glycophorin A from one individual with Cad+ red cells. They showed that in more than 71% of the side chains, the additional GalNAc residue had been added. It was also found[46] that the pentasaccharide that includes the Cad determinant is a potent inhibitor of anti-Sd^a. However, it is not clear whether this means that Cad and Sd^a are the same thing or whether a concentrated isolate of a structure similar to Sd^a, with GalNAc as the terminal residue, had the ability to cross-react with anti-Sd^a.

As an aside to descriptions of the fine structure of the molecules that include the Cad antigen, it can be added that Cartron et al[48] have shown that presence of the pentasaccharide instead of the usual tetrasaccharide on Cad+ cells, affords considerable protection for those red cells against invasion by merozoites of *Plasmodium falciparum*, the parasite that causes the most severe form of malaria in man. That it is the usual tetrasaccharide to which the merozoites normally bind is also shown by the findings that Tn cells, which have side chains that lack the terminal NeuAc and Gal residues[49,50] and En(a–) red cells, which lack glycophorin A altogether[51,52] and thus have drastically reduced numbers of side chains (ie, just those on glycophorin B and other minor membrane components), are also more resistant to invasion than are normal [ie, En(a+), Cad–, Tn–] red cells.[48,53]

Figure 3-2 also serves to illustrate the role of GalNAc as the immunodominant carbohydrate of the Tn antigen. This time, instead of GalNAc being added, as in Sd^a and Cad, two carbohydrates, NeuAc and Gal,

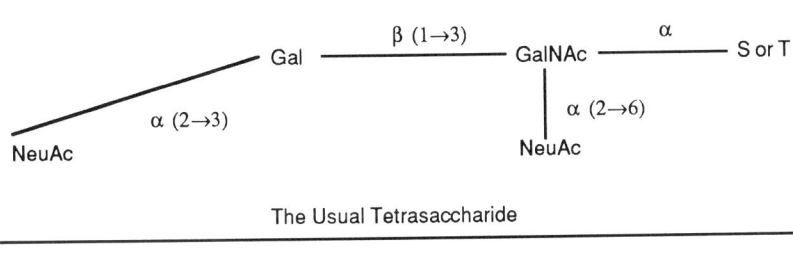

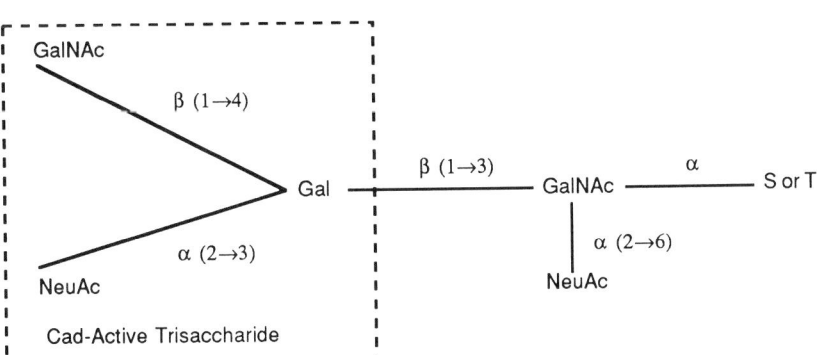

Figure 3-2. The usual, Cad-containing and Tn-containing oligosaccharides attached to (at least) glycophorin A. It is not clear whether the NeuAc in α(2→6) linkage to GalNAc is present in all, some or none Tn-containing structures. NeuAc = N-acetylneuraminic acid, Gal = D-galactose, GalNAc = N-acetyl-D-galactosamine, S = serine, T = threonine.

that are normally present in the tetrasaccharide are not added. Thus, a GalNAc residue that is normally present but not accessible (to antibody) is exposed on Tn-polyagglutinable red cells. As a second aside, the structures shown in Fig 3-2 (and others related to them) have been artificially synthesized.[54,55]

Are Sd^a and Cad the Same Antigen?

Clearly, at the serologic level, antigens that have GalNAc as their terminal immunodominant carbohydrate will display certain similarities. This is well-illustrated by the use of lectins. As mentioned earlier, the *D. biflorus* lectin recognizes both N-acetyl-α and β-D-galactosamine.[31] It agglutinates all red cells that carry enough copies of A (ie, it must be diluted for use as an anti-A_1 reagent so that it recognizes the quantitative difference in A antigen level on A_1 and A_2 red cells) and group O and B red cells that carry Tn or "super Sid" or Cad. Somewhat similarly, Tn-polyagglutinable red cells react more strongly with sera that contain anti-A than with those that do not.[56]

However, the specificity of a carbohydrate antigen is not wholly dependent on the terminal sugar residue. Serologic studies readily differentiate the specificities of anti-A, anti-P, anti-Tn and anti-Sd^a. The same is not true for anti-Sd^a and anti-Cad. In serologic studies, *D. biflorus* lectin agglutinates group O and group B Sd(a++) and Cad+ red cells (see Table 3-2 for the reactions of other lectins). Cad+ red cells react strongly with anti-Sd^a; that is, those with the highest level of Cad (Cad 1 and some Cad 2) behave as if they are Sd(a++).

What is not yet clear is whether these serologic findings represent identity between Sd^a and Cad as suggested,[6] or the presence of GalNAc in similar but not identical configurations in two slightly different antigens. If Sd^a and Cad are the same antigen, it would have to be supposed that *Sd^a* genes vary in a quantitative manner. That is to say, some would be highly efficient and their presence would result in the Sd(a++) or Cad+ phenotype. Others would appear to be less efficient and to vary in terms of the amount of Sd^a made. Since the *Sd^a* gene almost certainly encodes a galactosaminyltransferase, such an explanation would be entirely tenable. The situation would be very similar to that in which the transferases encoded by A^1, A^2, A^3, etc, result in different amounts of A antigen being present on red cells.

As discussed earlier, if Sd^a and Cad are the same, almost all Sd(a+) persons would have to be thought of as making some anti-Sd^a since the sera of almost all agglutinate polyagglutinable Cad 1 red cells. Again, the explanation is tenable since all persons with I+ red cells make low levels of clinically benign anti-I. However, a point in favor of thinking of Sd^a and Cad as the same is provided by a report[5] that the sera of persons with Sd(a++) red cells fail to agglutinate the polyagglutinable variety of Cad 1 red cells.

If Sd^a and Cad are, in fact, different antigens, it would have to be supposed that the *Sd^a* and *Cad* genes encode galactosaminyltransferases with slightly different specificities. If that is the case, the presence of anti-Cad in Sd(a+) and Sd(a−) persons would require no unusual explanation, and the antibodies would be regarded as being of universal incidence, as are anti-T, anti-Tn, anti-Tk, etc.

Naturally, it was hoped that recognition of the biochemical structure of Sd^a and Cad would answer the question of identity or nonidentity of the antigens. However, in this respect there is one highly important consideration that applies to the biochemical findings described above. While the structure of the Cad antigen on red cells is known, structural studies on Sd^a have, thus far, been confined to that antigen as present on the T-H urinary glycoprotein. It is not yet known if Sd^a has exactly the same structure when present on the red cell membrane. Duffy and Marshall[57] have pointed out that in the T-H glycoprotein there are carbohydrate side chains in N-linkage to five asparagine residues; at least two of these side chains are or include the Sd^a-containing pentasaccharide.[32,33] In contrast, on red cells, the pentasaccharides that include the Cad determinant are O-linked to threonine or serine.[46] There is only one N-linked-to-asparagine oligosaccharide on red cell glycophorin A.[58] As shown in Figs 3-1 and 3-2, the trisaccharides of Sd^a and Cad that inhibit human anti-Sd^a are the same. In the Sd^a-containing pentasaccharide, the trisaccharide is in $\beta(1 \rightarrow 4)$ linkage to GlcNAc. In the Cad-containing pentasaccharide, the trisaccharide is in $\beta(1 \rightarrow 3)$ linkage to GalNAc. However, again it must be remembered that the Sd^a-active structure represents Sd^a in the urine. It is not known to what or how the Sd^a-active trisaccharide is linked on red cells.

A different way in which the question about the identity or nonidentity of Sd^a and Cad might be answered would be to study the galactosaminyltransferases encoded by the Sd^a and Cad genes. Serafini-Cessi et al[39] isolated and purified the β-N-acetylgalactosaminyltransferase from the urine of individuals with Sd(a+) red cells. They found that the best acceptor for this enzyme, in its transfer of GalNAc in $\beta(1 \rightarrow 4)$ linkage to Gal, was a preparation of T-H glycoprotein isolated from the urine of an individual with Sd(a−) red cells. However, in its highly purified form (174-fold purification) the enzyme was also able to add GalNAc to the tetrasaccharides of native glycophorin A. The meaning of this observation is still not completely clear since Blanchard et al[46] did not find the additional GalNAc residue in the oligosaccharide side chains attached to glycophorin A of Sd(a+), Cad− red cells. Thus, it remains possible that the Sd^a-specified transferase may have preferential catalytic activity for N-linked oligosaccharides and the Cad-specified transferase preferential catalytic activity for O-linked oligosaccharides.

To summarize this long and somewhat tedious explanation, it will again be stated that the question used as a heading for this section may not be answered until the nature of the oligosaccharides that carry Sd^a on red cells is determined. While Sd^a and Cad on red cells may behave similarly in serologic studies, with "super Sid" and Cad appearing to be the same, that interpretation may or may not apply at the biochemical level. In other words, the current answer to the question that heads this section seems to be an unequivocal maybe!

References

1. Macvie SI, Morton JA, Pickles MM. The reactions and inheritance of a new blood group antigen, Sd[a]. Vox Sang 1967; 13:485-92.
2. Renton PH, Howell P, Ikin EW, et al. Anti-Sd[a], a new blood group antibody. Vox Sang 1967;13:493-501.
3. Lewis M, Anstee DJ, Bird GWG, et al. Blood group terminology 1990. Vox Sang 1990;58:152-69.
4. Morton JA, Pickles MM, Terry AM. The Sd[a] blood group antigen in tissues and body fluids. Vox Sang 1970;19:472-82.
5. Race RR, Sanger R. Blood groups in man. 6th ed. Oxford: Blackwell Scientific Publications, 1975:395-405.
6. Sanger R, Gavin J, Tippett P, et al. Plant agglutinin for another human blood-group. Lancet 1971;1:1130.
7. Sringarm S, Chupungart C, Giles CM. The use of *Ulex europaeus* and *Dolichos biflorus* extracts in routine ABO groupings of blood donors in Thailand. Vox Sang 1972;23:537-45.
8. Sringarm S, Chiewsilp P, Tubrod T. Cad receptors in Thai blood donors. Vox Sang 1974;26:462-6.
9. Pickles MM, Morton JA. The Sd[a] blood group. In: Mohn JF, Plunkett RW, Cunningham RK, Lambert RM, eds. Human blood groups. Basel: Karger, 1977:277-86.
10. Spitalnik S, Cox MT, Spennacchio J, et al. The serology of Sd[a] effects of transfusion and pregnancy. Vox Sang 1982;42: 308-12.
11. Howell P. Anti-Sd[a] and the blood group system it defines. Manchester: University of Manchester, 1968. Thesis.
12. Mollison PL, Engelfriet CP, Contreras M. Blood transfusion in clinical medicine. 8th ed. Oxford: Blackwell Scientific Publications, 1987: 400-1.
13. Silvergleid AJ, Wells RF, Hafleigh EB, et al. Compatibility test using [51]Chromium-labeled red blood cells in crossmatch positive patients. Transfusion 1978;18:8-14.
14. College KI, Kaplan HS, Marsh WL. Massive transfusion of Sd(a+) blood to a recipient with anti-Sd[a] without clinical complication (abstract). Transfusion 1973;13:340.
15. Peetermans ME, Cole-Dergent J. Haemolytic transfusion reaction due to anti-Sd[a]. Vox Sang 1970;18:67-70.
16. Lewis M, Kaita H, Chown B, et al. A family with the rare antigens Wr[a] and "super" Sd[a]. Vox Sang 1973;25:336-40.
17. Cazal P, Monis M, Caubel J, Brives J. Polyagglutinabilité héréditaire dominante: Antigène privé (Cad) correspondant à un anticorps public et à une lectine de *Dolichos biflorus*. Rev Fr Transf 1968;11:209-21.
18. Cazal P, Monis M, Bizot M. Les antigènes Cad et leurs rapports avec les antigènes A. Rev Fr Transf 1971;14:321-34.
19. Cazal P, Monis M, Bizot M. Les antigènes Cad en 1976. Rev Fr Transf Immunohematol 1977;20:165-73.

20. Crawford H, Cutbush M, Mollison PL. Specificity of incomplete "cold" antibody in human serum. Lancet 1953;1:566.
21. Issitt PD. Applied blood group serology. 3rd ed. Miami: Montgomery Scientific Publications, 1985.
22. Issitt PD, Jackson VA. Useful modifications and variations of technics in work on I system antibodies. Vox Sang 1968;15:152-3.
23. Anstee DJ. Blood group-active surface molecules of the human red blood cell. Vox Sang 1990;58:1-20.
24. Morton JA, Terry AM. The Sd^a blood group antigen. Biochemical properties of urinary Sd^a. Vox Sang 1970;19:151-61.
25. Morgan WTJ, Soh C, Watkins WM. Blood group Sd^a specificity as a possible genetic marker on Tamm and Horsfall urinary glycoprotein. In: Schauer R, Boer P, Buddecke E, et al, eds. Glycoconjugates. Stuttgart: Tieme Publishers, 1979:582-3.
26. Morgan WTJ, Soh CPC, Donald ASR, Watkins WM. Observations on the blood group Sd^a activity of Tamm and Horsfall urinary glycoprotein. Blood Transf Immunohaematol 1981;24:37-51.
27. Soh CPC, Morgan WTJ, Watkins WM, Donald ASR. The relationship between the N-acetylgalactosamine content and the blood group Sd^a activity of Tamm and Horsfall urinary glycoprotein. Biochem Biophys Res Comm 1980;93:1132-9.
28. Tamm I, Horsfall FL. Characterisation and separation of an inhibitor of viral haemagglutination present in urine. Proc Soc Exp Biol Med 1950;74:108-14.
29. Tamm I, Horsfall FL. A mucoprotein derived from human urine which reacts with influenza, mumps and Newcastle disease viruses. J Exp Med 1952;95:71-97.
30. Donald ASR, Soh CPC, Watkins WM, Morgan WTJ. N-acetyl-D-galactosaminyl-$\beta(1\rightarrow 4)$-D-galactose. A terminal non-reducing structure in human blood group Sd^a-active Tamm-Horsfall urinary glycoprotein. Biochem Biophys Res Comm 1982;104:58-65.
31. Hammarstrom S, Murphy LA, Goldstein IJ, Etzler ME. Carbohydrate binding specificity of four N-acetyl-D-galactosamine "specific" lectins: *Helix pomatia* A hemagglutinin, soy bean agglutinin, lima bean lectin and *Dolichos biflorus* lectin. Biochemistry 1977;16:2750-5.
32. Donald ASR, Yates AD, Soh CPC, et al. A blood group Sd^a-active pentasaccharide isolated from Tamm-Horsfall urinary glycoprotein. Biochem Biophys Res Comm 1983;115:625-31.
33. Williams J, Marshall RD, Van Halbeek H, Vliegenthart JFG. Structural analysis of the carbohydrate moieties of human Tamm-Horsfall glycoprotein. Carbohydr Res 1984;134:141-55.
34. Donald ASR, Yates AD, Soh CPC, et al. The human blood-group Sd^a determinant: A terminal non-reducing carbohydrate structure in N-linked and mucin-type glycoproteins. Biochem Soc Trans 1984;12:596-9.

35. Donald ASR, Feeney J. Oligosaccharides obtained from a blood-group-Sd(a+) Tamm-Horsfall glycoprotein. An n.m.r. study. Biochem J 1986;236:821-8.
36. Serafini-Cessi F, Dall'Olio F. Guinea-pig kidney β-N-acetyl-galactosaminyltransferase towards Tamm-Horsfall glycoprotein. Requirement of sialic acid in the acceptor for transferase activity. Biochem J 1983;215:483-9.
37. Donald ASR, Soh CPC, Yates AD, et al. Structure, biosynthesis and genetics of the Sd^a antigen. Biochem Soc Trans 1987;15:606-8.
38. Piller F, Blanchard D, Huet M, Cartron JP. Identification of a α-NeuAc(2→3)β-D-galactopyranosyl N-acetyl-β-D-galactosaminyltransferase in human kidney. Carbohydr Res 1986;149:171-84.
39. Serafini-Cessi F, Malagolini N, Dall'Olio F. Characterization and partial purification of β-N-acetylgalactosaminyltransferase from urine of Sd(a+) individuals. Arch Biochem Biophys 1988;266:573-82.
40. Schachter H, Michaels MA, Crookston MC, et al. A quantitative difference in the activity of blood group A-specific N-acetyl-galactosaminyltransferase in serum from A_1 and A_2 human subjects. Biochem Biophys Res Comm 1971;45:1011-18.
41. Tilley CA, Crookston MC, Crookston JH, et al. Human blood group *A*- and *H*-specified glycosyltransferase levels in the sera of newborn infants and their mothers. Vox Sang 1978;34:8-13.
42. Hammar L, Mannson S, Rohr T, et al. Lewis phenotypes of erythrocytes and Le^b-active glycolipid in serum of pregnant women. Vox Sang 1981;40:27-33.
43. Cartron JP, Blanchard D. Association of human erythrocyte membrane glycoproteins with blood-group Cad specificity. Biochem J 1982;207:497-504.
44. Bird GWG, Wingham J. Some serological properties of the Cad receptor. Vox Sang 1971;20:55-61.
45. Bird GWG, Wingham J. Hemagglutinins from *Salvia*. Vox Sang 1974; 26:163-6.
46. Blanchard D, Cartron JP, Fournet B, et al. Primary structure of the oligosaccharide determinant of blood group Cad specificity. J Biol Chem 1983;258:7691-5.
47. Herkt F, Parente JP, Leroy Y, et al. Structure determinations of oligosaccharides isolated from Cad erythrocyte membranes by permethylation analysis and 500-MHz ^{1}H-NMR spectroscopy. Eur J Biochem 1985;146:125-9.
48. Cartron JP, Prou O, Luilier M, Soulier JP. Susceptibility to invasion by *Plasmodium falciparum* of some human erythrocytes carrying rare blood group antigens. Br J Haematol 1983;55:639-47.
49. Dahr W, Uhlenbruck G, Bird GWG. Cryptic A-like receptor sites in human erythrocyte glycoproteins: Proposed nature of Tn-antigen. Vox Sang 1974;27:29-42.

50. Dahr W, Uhlenbruck G, Gunson HH, van der Hart M. Studies on glycoproteins and glycopeptides from Tn-polyagglutinable erythrocytes. Vox Sang 1975;28:249-52.
51. Dahr W, Uhlenbruck G, Leikola J, et al. Studies on the membrane glycoprotein defect of En(a–) erythrocytes. I. Biochemical aspects. J Immunogenet 1976;3:329-46.
52. Tanner MJA, Anstee DJ. The membrane change in En(a–) human erythrocytes. Biochem J 1976;153:271-7.
53. Pasvol G, Wainscoat JS, Weatherall DJ. Erythrocytes deficient in glycophorin resist invasion by the malarial parasite *Plasmodium falciparum*. Nature 1982;297:64-6.
54. Catelani G, Marra A, Paquet F, Sinay P. Chemical synthesis of the desialylated human Cad-antigenic determinant. Carbohydr Res 1986; 155:131-40.
55. Marra A, Sinay P. Synthesis of sialylated branched tri- and tetra-saccharide derivatives with the sequence of the Cad blood group determinant. Gazz Chim Ital 1987;117:563-6.
56. Berman HJ, Smarto J, Issitt CH, et al. Tn-activation with an acquired A-like antigen. Transfusion 1972;12:35-45.
57. Duffy FA, Marshall RD. The immunological, genetic and biosynthetic relationships of the Cad and Sd^a antigens. Biochem Soc Trans 1985; 13:1128-9.
58. Marchesi VT, Furthmayr H, Tomita M. The red cell membrane. Ann Rev Biochem 1976;45:667-98.

In: Moulds JM and Woods LL, eds.
Blood Groups: P, I, Sd^a and Pr
Arlington, VA: American Association of Blood Banks, 1991

4

Cold-Reactive Autoantibodies Outside the I and P Blood Groups

Peter D. Issitt, PhD, FIMLS, FIBiol, CBiol, FRCPath

AS DISCUSSED IN DETAIL in Chapter 2 of this book, most cases of cold hemagglutinin disease (CHD, CHAD, also called "cold" antibody-induced hemolytic anemia) are caused by autoantibodies of the I blood group. As described in Chapter 1, paroxysmal cold hemoglobinuria (PCH) is caused by an autoreactive, biphasic hemolysin with anti-P specificity. However, many other cold-reactive autoantibodies with different specificities (and names) have been recognized. Often these antibodies were first studied because they caused (sometimes severe) "cold" antibody-induced hemolytic anemia. In a few instances, after the specificities had been recognized and partially characterized, benign forms of the same specificity were found. This chapter attempts to list these antibodies and to describe them and the antigens they define, in terms of what is known at the serologic, immunologic, clinical and biochemical levels. Because of the fact that so many of these autoantibodies were first found when they caused CHD, frequent mention of that fact will be made. However, it should be borne in mind that if all cases of CHD caused by other than I blood group antibodies are added together, they still comprise a small minority of the total cases.

The Pr Antigens

In 1968, Marsh and Jenkins[1] described several examples of a cold-reactive autoantibody that caused severe CHD in some of the subjects studied. In tests on samples from thousands of normal donors, no nonreactive red cells were found. The antibodies clearly differed from those of the I blood

---

Peter D. Issitt, PhD, FIMLS, FIBiol, CBiol, FRCPath, Associate Professor of Pathology and Scientific Director, Immunohematology, Transfusion Service, Duke University Medical Center, Durham, North Carolina

group; red cells from adults and from cord blood samples reacted to about the same degree (using undiluted sera and in titrations) and the antigen(s) defined was (were) denatured when red cells were treated with ficin. The authors pointed out that lack of a nonreactive blood sample meant that while they could describe the antibodies as similar and likely to be related, they could not be certain that all examples defined the same antigen. Such a conclusion was prophetic; as described below, the fine specificities of these antibodies have enabled recognition of a large number of antigens. Marsh and Jenkins[1] assigned the name anti-Sp_1 to the new antibody. The Sp was an abbreviation for species (since the red cells of all humans were reactive) and the subscript was used to characterize the first antibody; allowance was already being made for the many specificities now known. In fact, the terms Sp_2, Sp_3 etc, did not become widely used; instead, the change in terminology described below took place.

At about the same time as the work on Sp_1 was being done in England, autoantibodies of ostensibly similar specificity were being studied in Germany. When they published their initial findings, Roelcke and Dorrow[2] called the antibody anti-HD, after Heidelberg, the city in which the study was performed. However, a comment was published[3] to the effect that the term HD might be taken to imply that the antigen was present only on red cells that carried both H and D. This led Roelcke and Uhlenbruck[4] to suggest that the terms Sp_1, HD_1 and HD_2 be replaced by Pr_1 and Pr_2. The Pr was derived from protease, since by then it was known[1,5-10] that more than one antigen was involved, that all the antigens were protease-sensitive and that at least some of the antigens were destroyed (or removed) when red cells were treated with neuraminidase. The name Pr was said to be more suitable than Sp since it had also been shown[1,4-6,10] that the antigens were present on the red cells of many species in addition to man. At this point it should be added that while these antigens are removed from human red cells when those cells are treated with protease, the same is not true of red cells from other species. As discussed in detail below, some Pr antibodies give markedly enhanced reactions when tested against protease-treated red cells from dogs.

Following these initial studies, an enormous amount of work was done at the serologic and biochemical levels on the Pr antigens and antibodies, much of it in the laboratories of Dr. Dieter Roelcke in Heidelberg. Brief synopses of many of the findings are given below. Extensive references are provided for those readers who wish to consult the original papers that presented the results from which the conclusions given were drawn.

Serology of the Pr Antigens and Antibodies

1. The red cells of almost all humans react equally with anti-Pr of different specificities. There are no Pr equivalents to the I adult, i adult and i cord phenotypes. All Pr activity of human red cells is lost

when those cells are treated with papain, ficin or bromelin. All Pr activity on human red cells, except Pr_a, is lost when the red cells are treated with neuraminidase. To take advantage of this fact in antibody identification studies, anti-T must be removed from the sera under test, by adsorption. Red cells that are devoid of MN sialoglycoprotein (SGP) [eg, En(a–) or from M^k homozygotes] may give weak or negative reactions in direct tests with anti-Pr. Red cells with reduced numbers of copies and/or markedly altered MN SGP (eg, from Mi^V homozygotes) may give weaker reactions than normal red cells with anti-Pr. For an explanation of these findings see the section on biochemistry.

2. The Pr antigens have been divided into those now called Pr_1, Pr_2, Pr_3, Pr_a, Pr^M (and probably Pr^N). The initial division between Pr_1 and Pr_2 was that the Pr_1 antigen as defined by some antibodies was found on human but not dog red cells. Although other examples of anti-Pr_1 did react with dog red cells (for this subdivision see below) that reaction was abolished when the dog cells were treated with a protease. Anti-Pr_2 reacted strongly with untreated but not with protease-treated human red cells; it reacted with dog red cells, that reaction being enhanced when such cells were protease-treated.[11] Pr_3 was differentiated from Pr_1 and Pr_2 when it was found on the red cells of cats and sheep; both species have red cells that lack Pr_1 and Pr_2.[12] Differences between Pr_1, Pr_2 and Pr_3 have also been found at the biochemical level (see below). Such findings have very clearly authenticated that different antigens are involved and have illustrated how perceptive were the conclusions drawn from the serologic studies.[11-15] The antigens Pr_a, Pr^M and the putative Pr^N were differentiated later and are described below.

3. The antigens Pr_1 and Pr_3 have now both been subdivided. Pr_{1h} and Pr_{3h} are found on human but not dog red cells. Pr_{1d} and Pr_{3d} are found on both human and dog red cells.[10-13] As mentioned above, all examples of anti-Pr_2 have reacted with dog red cells.[13,16,17]

4. For details of 13 breeds of dogs whose red cells have been tested for the presence of Pr_{1d} and/or Pr_{3d}, see reference 11.

5. Humans and dogs are not the only species whose red cells carry Pr antigens. Various different publications[12,13,16-19] have described the presence of some of the antigens (see Table 4-1) on the red cells of guinea pigs, rats, sheep and cats. Some of the antigens have also been found on the tissue cells of guinea pigs and rats.[20]

6. The antigens Pr_1, Pr_2 and Pr_3 are also destroyed or denatured when red cells are treated with neuraminidase.[5,8,12,13,16,17] In order to demonstrate this fact, it is necessary to adsorb anti-T (that reacts with neuraminidase-treated T-activated red cells) from the sera containing anti-Pr.

7. When anti-Pr_a was first named,[21] it was said to define an antigen that was removed when red cells were treated with protease, but that

Table 4-1. The Most Typical Reactions of Anti-Pr Subspecificities*

Red Cells	Pr$_{1h}$	Pr$_{1d}$	Pr$_2$	Pr$_{3h}$	Pr$_{3d}$	Pr$_a$	Pr^M	Pr^N
I$_{Adult}$								
Unttd	+	+	+	+	+	+	+s	+=
Prot	0	0	0	0	0	0	0	0
Nmdase	0	0	0	0	0	+	0	0
i$_{Adult}$								
Unttd	+	+	+	+	+	+	+s	+=
Prot	0	0	0	0	0	0	0	0
Nmdase	0	0	0	0	0	+	0	0
i$_{cord}$								
Unttd	+	+	+	+	+	+	+s	+=
Prot	0	0	0	0	0	0	0	0
Nmdase	0	0	0	0	0	+	0	0

Dog					
Unttd	0	0	0	0	0
Prot	0	+†	+ E	0	0
Nmdase	0	V 0	0	0	0
Sheep	0	0	0	0	+
Cat	0	0	0	0	+
Guinea Pig	V	V	+		E
Rat	V	V	V		V
Rabbit‖	0	0	0	0	0

*The most usual reactions are shown. For exceptions see text and references given therein.

†Some anti-Pr$_{1d}$ react only weakly with dog red cells.

§Reactions of all cells equal in tests at low (4 C) temperatures. Reactions of M+ cells stronger than those of M− red cells in tests at higher (20–25 C) temperatures.

‖Similar to note above except that preference is for N+ cells.

¶Red cells from rabbits are useful in differential adsorption studies since they lack the Pr determinants but carry I and i.

Unttd = untreated, Prot = protease-treated, Nmdase = neuraminidase-treated, + = agglutination, V = variable reaction, ie, some negative, some positive. In titration studies, cells marked V usually react to a lower titer than those marked +. E = enhanced reaction. In titration studies, cells marked E usually react to higher titers than those marked +. Blank spaces = no information available.

remained detectable on neuraminidase-treated red cells. When the original antibody was reinvestigated[22] it was shown that it was anti-T in the serum that was responsible for the reaction with the neuraminidase-treated red cells. However, Habibi et al[23] found an antibody in a newborn that fit the criteria established[21] for anti-Pr_a specificity. Thus, Pr_a differs from Pr_1, Pr_2 and Pr_3 in that it is detectable on neuraminidase-treated red cells. As with all Pr antigens, Pr_a is denatured by protease treatment of red cells.

8. As described in some detail in the section on biochemistry of the Pr antigens, those determinants are known to reside in some oligosaccharide side chains attached to the MN, Ss and other sialoglycoproteins. However, Pr_1, Pr_2, Pr_3 and Pr_a are not dependent on the presence of M or N for reactivity. In contrast, anti-Pr^M behaves much like other examples of anti-Pr in tests at low temperatures (ie, it reacts equally well with M+N− and M−N+ red cells) but shows a distinct preference for M+ red cells in tests at higher temperatures.[24] In other words, the Pr^M determinant is influenced by the amino acid sequence of glycophorin A[25] and in that respect differs from Pr_1, Pr_2, Pr_3 and Pr_a. An antibody that Roelcke[17] suggests probably had anti-Pr^N specificity was described earlier[26] but that name was not used.

9. Autoantibodies directed against the Pr determinants may be IgM,[1,13,16,17,24,27-35] IgG[21,36-39] or IgA[2,40-43] in nature. In reviewing reports about a large number of cold-reactive autoantibodies and in comparing the findings to those in his own laboratory, Roelcke[17] pointed out that among IgM autoantibodies with kappa light chains, all specificities are found but anti-I predominates by far. IgM autoantibodies with lambda light chains are more likely to have specificity outside the I blood group; Pr antibodies are often included. Roelcke[17] also pointed out that all published examples of pathologic IgA cold agglutinins had Pr specificity and wondered if their preponderance in this group denotes a restriction in the immune response mechanism. As discussed in more detail below, many of the Pr-specific autoantibodies found (as with other specificity autoantibodies causative of CHD) have been monoclonal in nature.

10. While most cases of autoantibody-induced hemolytic anemia caused by anti-Pr have been, or have closely resembled CHD, a few, particularly when the anti-Pr was IgG, have had some similarities to "warm" antibody-induced hemolytic anemia. The case described by McGinniss et al[37] involved a "warm" reactive IgG autoanti-Pr_a. That patient had a purine nucleoside phosphorylase deficiency and when the authors found a similar antibody in another patient with that disorder, they suggested that the two conditions might, in some way, be related. The patient described by Curtis et al[39] had life-threatening hemolytic anemia and failed to respond to conventional drug therapy. His autoantibody was an IgG1 anti-Pr_a and his hemolytic anemia

was resolved by splenectomy. Mechanisms of red cell clearance by anti-Pr are discussed again, below.

11. In classic PCH a biphasic hemolysin (the D-L or Donath-Landsteiner antibody) that almost always has anti-P specificity[44,45] causes sudden acute episodes of red cell hemolysis that lead to hemoglobinuria. Episodes of hemolysis are precipitated by exposure of the patient to cold temperatures. However, not all D-L biphasic hemolysins cause PCH. In some cases there is no hemoglobinuria and hemolysis is neither episodic nor precipitated by cold exposure. Such cases are most accurately described as D-L hemolytic anemia.[46] One case has been documented in which the D-L type autoantibody had anti-Pr specificity.[47]

12. Most examples of autoanti-Pr are causative of CHD. While it was typical in this respect, an IgM anti-Pr_{1d} described by Green et al[48] was unique in that it was inhibited by sodium citrate. Indeed, when unwashed red cells in preservatives were used for testing, the cold agglutinin appeared too weak to be of clinical significance. When it was titrated against washed red cells, its titer was greater than 2000. Examples of autoanti-Pr not causing CHD have been reported.[18,19,23,49] However, in several of these patients, C3 was found on the red cells when DATs were performed. In the case reported by Bell et al[49] there was evidence that transfused red cells did not enjoy normal in vivo survival although no clinical signs of a transfusion reaction were noted when the patient was transfused with blood passed through a warming coil. Two patients described by O'Neill et al[50] had anti-Pr_1 reactive only in tests performed at low ionic strength. Again, there was no evidence for CHD and transfusions were uneventful, but both patients had positive DATs with C3 on their red cells.

13. In an earlier review[25] of Pr specificities, two forms of anti-Pr_3 were listed. It is now known[17] that the anti-Pr_3 described by Roelcke et al[12] was an example of anti-Pr_{3d}, while that described by Birgens et al[18] was the first example of anti-Pr_{3h}. An antibody described by Roelcke et al[19] that was listed as anti-Pr Ad in the earlier review[25] now seems to have been classified[17] as a somewhat atypical form of anti-Pr_{1d}. Roelcke[17] notes that Pr_{1d} may be completely or partially inactivated when dog red cells are treated with proteases.

Biochemistry of the Pr Antigens

Pr_1, Pr_2 and Pr_3

The early finding that protease-treated red cells do not react with anti-Pr clearly indicated that the antigens are carried on protease-sensitive components of the red cell membrane. The finding that most anti-Pr do not react with neuraminidase-treated red cells showed that neuraminic acid, which is specifically cleaved when red cells are treated with neuraminidase, must be an integral part of the antigens. Thus, it was not too surprising to learn[16,51-53] that when extracts are made from red cell membranes in such a way that they include glycophorin A (the MN SGP), those extracts have the ability to inhibit anti-Pr_1, -Pr_2 and -Pr_3. Glycophorin A carries up to 15 copies of the tetrasaccharide side chain depicted in Fig 4-1.[54-56] The term "up to 15 copies" is used since it is now known that on the portion of the SGP closest to the red cell membrane, some of the side chains are trisaccharides that lack one or the other of the N-acetylneuraminic acid (NeuAc) residues. Liskowska et al[56] have shown that on most red cells, the ratio of tetrasaccharides to trisaccharides (Fig 4-1) lacking the $\alpha(2\rightarrow6)$ linked NeuAc, to trisaccharides lacking the $\beta(1\rightarrow3)$ linked NeuAc, is 8:3:1. Dahr[57] has shown that glycophorin B (the Ss SGP) that also carries copies of the tetrasaccharide is Pr_1-, Pr_2- and Pr_3-active.

As discussed below, it is possible that the Pr determinants are also present on minor red cell SGPs and perhaps other membrane structures. The Pr_1, Pr_2 and Pr_3 determinants are carried wholly within the tetrasac-

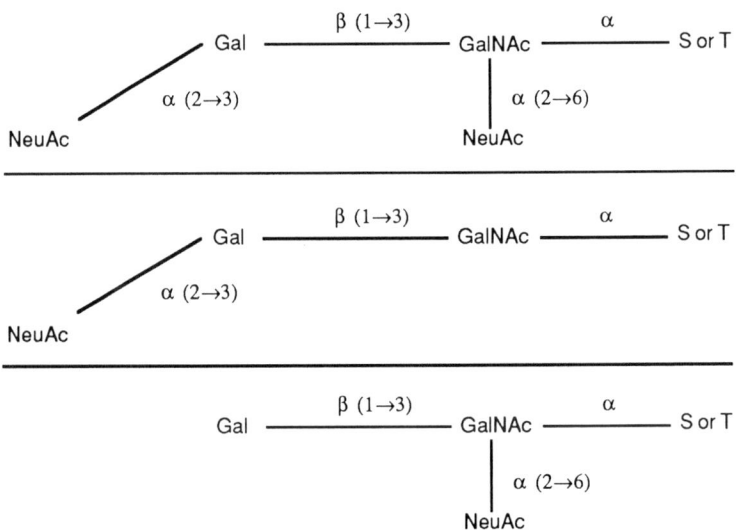

Figure 4-1. The structures of a tetrasaccharide and two trisaccharides bound to human glycophorins. NeuAc = N-acetylneuraminic acid, Gal = D-galactose, GalNAc = N-acetyl-D-galactosamine, S = serine, T = threonine.

charide shown in Fig 4-1. That is to say, the MN polymorphism that results from different amino acids at positions one and five at the NH_2 terminal end of the protein backbone of the MN SGP (for a review see reference 25), plays no role in the structure of these antigens. When the tetrasaccharides are isolated from the protein backbones of the SGPs, they retain Pr activity.[58] While it is clear that the Pr determinants are carried within the tetrasaccharide of Fig 4-1, it is not yet known which portions of that structure comprise which antigens nor whether both NeuAc residues are essential for antigen integrity. There are conflicting reports on the inhibition of Pr antibodies using NeuAc alone. Roelcke and Kreft[16] used NeuAc at concentrations of up to 20 mmol/L (6.2 mg/mL) but saw no inhibition of any anti-Pr in their collection. In contrast, Garratty and O'Neill[59] found five anti-Pr that were inhibited using NeuAc at concentrations from 1 to 10 mg/mL; the two LISS-dependent anti-Pr that those workers[50] reported were not inhibited.

Different inhibition and enhancement patterns, closely correlated to anti-Pr subspecificities, were seen when chemically modified preparations of isolated glycophorins that included tetrasaccharides were used. When such extracts are periodate-oxidized the trihydroxyside chain of NeuAc is shortened, creating a C7 NeuAc derivate.[60] Carbodiimide treatment of the glycophorin extracts may cause an N-acyl-urea derivative of NeuAc, which is formed by rearrangement from an O-acyl-urea derivative of NeuAc after reaction with the carboxy group of NeuAc.[61] Both periodate oxidation and carbodiimide treatment destroyed Pr_1 activity. For Pr_2, periodate oxidation increased activity some 100 to 200-fold; carbodiimide treatment destroyed it. For Pr_3 the effects were exactly the reverse of those on Pr_2. Periodate oxidation destroyed Pr_3 activity, while carbodiimide treatment increased it some 100- to 200-fold.[12,53,62,63] As mentioned earlier, these findings at the biochemical level were a triumphant endorsement of the Pr_1, Pr_2 and Pr_3 subdivisions made earlier at the serologic level. These findings, expressed in terms of enhancement or destruction of Pr antigen activity, are summarized in Table 4-2.

As will by now be clear, distinct differences between Pr_1, Pr_2 and Pr_3 exist at the biochemical level. To these can be added the observation that of the three determinants, Pr_2 alone appears to be present on gangliosides and other lipids.[64,65] As mentioned in the section on the serology of Pr, Pr_2 is still detectable on protease-treated dog red cells. These two observations have led Roelcke[17] to suggest that perhaps on dog red cells, Pr_2 is restricted to gangliosides. That the same is not true of human red cells is clear from the findings that Pr_2 is denatured when such red cells are treated with protease and that glycophorin preparations from human red cells are Pr_2-active. Thus, it seems unlikely that ganglioside-borne Pr_2 contributes significantly to the reaction between human red cells and anti-Pr_2.

Table 4-2. Inhibition and Enhancement of Anti-Pr Using Unaltered and Chemically Modified Oligosaccharides Derived from Human Red Cell Glycophorins

Antibody	Unttd*	Human Red Cell Glycoproteins Oxid‡	Carbod§
Anti-Pr_{1h}	+	0	0[∥]
Anti-Pr_{1d}	+	0	0[∥]
Anti-Pr_2	+	+ ↑	0
Anti-Pr_{3h}	+	0	+ ↑
Anti-Pr_{3d}	+	0	+ ↑
Anti-Pr_a	+		

*Untreated glycophorin extracts.
‡Periodate-oxidized glycophorin extracts.
§Carbodiimide-treated glycophorin extracts.
+ = antibody inhibition, 0 = no antibody inhibition, + ↑ = inhibitory effect increased 100 to 200 fold, $0^{\parallel}$ = some anti-Pr_1 partially inhibited.

Pr_a

Based on serologic observations, it would seem that Pr_a must have a fundamentally different biochemical structure to the Pr_1, Pr_2 and Pr_3 antigens. Anti-Pr_a fails to react with protease-treated human red cells; it does react with such cells treated with neuraminidase. Thus, while Pr_a (as with Pr_1, Pr_2 and Pr_3) would appear to be carried on a protease-sensitive red cell membrane component, it would seem not to require NeuAc for its structural integrity. However, Roelcke and Kreft[16] found that one anti-Pr_a in their collection was strongly inhibited with chemically modified glycophorin extracts (see above), while a second example was not. This finding would seem to suggest two possibilities. First, not all antibodies called anti-Pr_a may have exactly the same specificity. Second, since the modifications to the glycophorin preparations should have altered only sialyl groups, perhaps one form of anti-Pr_a defines a determinant that includes one or more neuraminidase (sialidase) insensitive NeuAc residues on glycophorins. Given the already well-established subdivisions of Pr_1 and Pr_3, it would not be at all surprising to find that Pr_a can be subdivided (remember, you read it here, first!).

Pr^M, Pr^N

Anti-Pr^M reacts strongly with all red cells when tests are performed at low (ie, refrigerator) temperatures. In tests at warmer (ie, ambient) temperatures the antibody shows a distinct preference for red cells that carry M.

It is well-known that at different temperatures red cell membrane structures assume slightly different three-dimensional shapes. Thus, it is not difficult to imagine that at 4 C the Pr^M antigen can be recognized in any glycophorin A-bound tetrasaccharide. At higher temperatures it seems that the amino acids at positions one and five on the M gene-specified SGP contribute to orientation of the tetrasaccharides and hence the three-dimensional shape of Pr^M. Inhibition studies support this assumption entirely. Anti-Pr^M can be inhibited by any glycophorin extract. It is preferentially inhibited by fragments linked to the *M* gene-specified protein backbone.[24] An antibody described by Hinz and Boyer[26] was not fully characterized at the serologic level (it was described before the Pr antigens had been studied and named) but was somewhat analogous to anti-Pr^M in its reactivity. That is to say, at low temperatures the antibody reacted with all cells; at warmer temperatures it showed a distinct preference for those that were N+. In retrospect it seems that the suggestion[17] that this antibody had anti-Pr^N specificity is entirely justified.

Other Possible Sites of Pr Determinants

Anstee[66] has suggested that the Pr determinants are present in oligosaccharides within the area of the amino-terminal 26 residues of those SGPs. However, adsorption studies and some observations cited below seem to suggest that while the outer portions of the SGPs carry the number of copies of Pr determinants necessary for red cells to be agglutinated by anti-Pr, a smaller number of copies may well be present in oligosaccharides attached to the more internal portions of glycophorins A and B. Dahr[67] has pointed out that the minor red cell sialoglycoproteins (glycophorins C, D etc) are also glycosylated and may well carry tetrasaccharides or similar structures that include Pr determinants.

At both the serologic and biochemical levels, proving this point is difficult because of the paucity of copies of the minor SGPs as compared to glycophorins A and B. Indeed, similar considerations may well apply to nonglycophorin glycosylated red cell membrane components that may include structures that carry Pr. The finding that protease-treated red cells no longer react with anti-Pr does not contradict the suggestion that some Pr determinants may be present on red cell membrane components other than glycophorins A and B. Indeed, under some circumstances protease-treatment of red cells does not effect total cleavage of glycophorin B. Further, some protease-resistant minor red cell membrane structures may carry a few Pr determinants.

Thus, the apparent conversion from the Pr+ to the Pr− state, by treatment of red cells with proteases, may simply reflect a quantitative difference in the number of available Pr receptors on red cells with glycophorin A present and those (protease-treated) from which most of the structure has been removed. It is not yet known whether or not red cells from M^k

homozygotes, which lack all expression of glycophorins A and B,[68] carry Pr antigens.

Differentiation Between Anti-Pr and Anti-En^a

As discussed in detail in the previous section, the vast majority of Pr determinants on human red cells are carried in oligosaccharide side chains attached to glycophorin A. Other Pr determinants are present in identical side chains attached to glycophorin B. However, because red cells have, on average, some five times more copies of glycophorin A than of glycophorin B and because each copy of glycophorin A carries many more side chains than each copy of glycophorin B, the major site of Pr determinants (ie, number of copies) is glycophorin A. As mentioned above, glycophorins C, D and other structures would contribute even fewer copies. Thus, En(a–) red cells, which lack glycophorin A,[69-71] have a markedly reduced number of copies of Pr determinants. This means that in antibody identification studies, anti-Pr may fail to react with En(a–) red cells and may be mistaken for anti-En^a. In fact, the lack of reaction between anti-Pr and En(a–) red cells represents the presence of too few antigens on the cells to support agglutination, not lack of the antigen that the antibody defines.

Serologic studies against protease-treated red cells will not always differentiate between anti-Pr and anti-En^a. While such treated cells will have lost their serologically recognizable Pr determinants, they will also have lost two of the three known En^a antigens, En^{a}TS and En^{a}FS. Only anti-En^{a}FR will continue to react with protease-treated red cells.[72] When we[73] first encountered the phenomenon of anti-Pr failing to react with En(a–) red cells, we reasoned that those cells should carry enough copies of the Pr determinants to be able to adsorb the antibody; this, indeed, proved to be the case. En(a–) cells will not, of course, adsorb antibodies directed against En^{a}TS, En^{a}FS or En^{a}FR. An identical adsorption procedure was later used by McGinniss et al[37] for the same purpose. Homberg et al[74] succeeded in making anti-Pr agglutinate En(a–) red cells by performing tests in a system adjusted to pH 6.2.

The study by Brunt and Vengelen-Tyler,[75] in which it was shown that many examples of anti-Pr reacted poorly with red cells with no or with altered MN SGP, clearly related to the number of copies of Pr determinants on the test red cells. Red cells that are S–s–U– have been shown[76-78] to lack glycophorin B, so carry fewer copies of the Pr determinants than do red cells that carry glycophorins A and B. However, such is the profusion of Pr determinants on glycophorin A, that is expressed normally on S–s–U– cells, that we[25] have not been able to demonstrate any weakening of Pr antigen expression on those cells.

When they studied two brothers who were homozygous for M^k, Tokunga et al[68] described a "naturally occurring" antibody in one of them that was almost certainly anti-Pr. Unfortunately, no adsorption studies using the red cells of these individuals and anti-Pr were reported. Certainly, if red cells from M^k homozygotes, which lack glycophorins A and B, had been shown capable of adsorbing even limited amounts of anti-Pr, it would have shown that Pr determinants are carried (albeit in low site density) on red cell membrane structures other than glycophorins A and B.

The Pr Antibodies: Some Immunologic Considerations

As already mentioned, many examples of anti-Pr have been shown to be causative of hemolytic anemia, usually but not always of the "cold" antibody type. Like cases caused by other cold-reactive autoantibodies, those caused by anti-Pr can be divided into two broad general categories. First are those hemolytic episodes, often transient in nature, that follow infections. Second are cases of chronic CHD that represent proliferation of an aberrant clone of immunocytes. In cases of hemolytic anemia caused by anti-Pr, the former seem more common (albeit still unusual)[12,14,16,17,21,38,39,42,43,47] than the latter.[1,6,13,14,24,42,48,79,80] In cases in which infections, such as those caused by *Mycoplasma pneumoniae*, Epstein-Barr virus (EBV), rubella virus (that seems[17] particularly prone to stimulate production of anti-Pr), varicella, cytomegalovirus and other viruses (including unidentified ones that cause acute febrile illnesses), are followed by transient hemolytic episodes, there are three possible explanations.

First, it is possible that the antibodies that destroy the red cells are actually directed against the infectious agent, are produced as a response to the infection and cross-react with red cell surface antigens. However, evidence for shared or similar immunogenic structures on the infectious agents and red cells is lacking.

Second, it is possible that anti-idiotypes or even anti-anti-idiotypes, produced to control production of antibodies against the infectious agents, find mirror image determinants on red cells and are thus able to complex with and destroy those cells.

Third, it is possible that the infectious agents somehow disrupt T-cell regulation of B cells and allow otherwise "forbidden clones" of immunocytes to make autoantibody.

Little is known about the etiology of chronic CHD. When antibodies to Pr are produced, the disorder may be associated with lymphoproliferative disease or lymphoma, or may occur in individuals without other discernable clinical abnormalities.[26,28,29,31,33,34] This, of course, is no different from chronic CHD caused by autoantibodies other than anti-Pr. It is known[81] that Pr determinants are present on the membranes of macrophages and of T and B cells. However, it is not known how this observation relates to the production of pathologic autoantibodies in primary or secondary CHD. Among cold-reactive autoagglutinins of all specificities, causative of CHD, the majority are monoclonal in nature. This finding certainly applies to pathologic autoanti-Pr whether the antibody is produced following infection or in chronic CHD.[13,16,17,24,31,33,34,36,38,39,43,79,80]

Roelcke[17] has suggested that the production of monoclonal cold autoagglutinins may be a two-step procedure. In the first step, it is suggested that an infectious agent renders host or self antigens immunogenic. In the second step, production of the cold agglutinin may become chronic by a combined process of Ig isotype translocation with concomitant oncogene activation. It is, of course, entirely possible that in the chronic form of the disease, the initial triggering event occurs during an infection. Perhaps the difference between chronic CHD and the transient hemolytic episodes that follow recent infection is that in the former, once autoantibody production is started, it cannot be regulated by the immune system. The pathologic clone of immunocytes proliferates and autoantibody production becomes permanent, thus causing chronic disease. Perhaps in the transient hemolytic episodes, the abnormal immunocytes can be regulated ("switched off") by the immune system so that autoantibody production is transient and the episodes of hemolysis self-limiting; that is, they do not continue because autoantibody production is curtailed.

As mentioned earlier, there are some indications that production of monoclonal, pathologic cold-reactive autoantibodies is more likely to be a function of, or may be restricted to, certain clones of immunocytes. For example, most but not quite all, pathologic autoanti-I are IgM molecules with kappa light chains. Exceptions have been reported.[27,30,82,83] While many anti-i are IgM antibodies with kappa light chains, a higher proportion of anti-i than of anti-I are IgM with lambda light chains. In this respect autoanti-Pr are somewhat heterogeneous. References are given above describing autoanti-Pr that were IgM, IgG and IgA. However, when 36 anti-Pr were studied in one laboratory,[16] 31 were IgM, four IgA and one IgG. Among 19 of the antibodies typed for light chain type, 18 had kappa and one had lambda light chains. While autoanti-Pr may be of any immunoglobulin type (with IgM predominating), IgA cold-reactive autoantibodies that actually cause CHD may all have anti-Pr specificity. Roelcke[17] has suggested that this may possibly represent a restriction of pathologic IgA cold autoantibodies to Pr specificities. While Ratkin et al[84] and Hsu et al[85] have presented evidence that many persons who make pathologic IgM anti-I, make small amounts of IgG and IgA anti-I as well, the IgG and IgA antibodies in those patients may not have contributed to the immune red cell destruction. A recently reported case[86] in which a patient made IgM and IgA anti-I was unique in that the patient had a biclonal gammopathy.

Idiotypes

Because monoclonal cold agglutinins have distinct specificities, it would be hoped that those of the same specificity might share idiotypes. The idiotype of an antibody represents the arrangement of amino acids, ie, a structural region, within the antigen-binding site of the antibody molecules. Antibodies against idiotypes can be raised in animals,[87,88] by using hybridoma technology[89] or by EBV transformation of B cells.[90] However, the use of anti-idiotypes to study cold agglutinins is not as straightforward as the above, somewhat simplistic, definition might imply. For example, while some anti-idiotypes raised against Pr antibodies did define idiotypes shared by different examples of the antibodies[80,87] and some were shown[87,88] not to cross-react with anti-I or anti-i, others, raised against I system cold agglutinins, were shown[91,92] to react with some paraproteins that were not antibodies to red cell antigens. In other cases[93-95] anti-idiotypes have been quite individualistic and have reacted only with the antibody against which they were raised.

Silberstein et al[96] used EBV transformation of B cells from a patient with a pathologic anti-Pr_2 in the serum to produce a series of clones of cells secreting anti-Pr_2. Jefferies et al[95] then used cells from those clones to immunize mice whose spleen cells were later fused with a mouse myeloma cell line and monoclonal anti-idiotype specificities were obtained. Two of the anti-idiotypes were IgG1, two were IgM and all four had kappa light chains. Inhibition experiments suggested that the four anti-idiotypes were directed against identical or neighboring idiotypes on the anti-Pr_2 molecules, both heavy and light chains of those molecules were necessary for idiotype integrity, but the anti-idiotypes did not combine with anti-Pr other than that of the original patient.[96] The authors[95] pointed out that anti-idiotypes produced against B-cell lymphomas, in which no red cell autoantibodies were being made, also appeared to be tumor specific.[97]

As discussed in Chapter 2 and as mentioned briefly above, more progress has been made in studying anti-idiotype specificities directed against anti-I cold agglutinins than in studying those directed against anti-Pr. Clearly, work on anti-idiotypes to cold agglutinins has two highly important objectives. First, their use may help to answer the question as to which clones produce monoclonal autoantibodies and provide information as to the nature of the defect that results in activation of those clones. Second, the anti-idiotypes may be of value in immunotherapy either by neutralizing the pathologic cold agglutinins in vivo or by curtailing their production. Indeed, clinical trials using anti-idiotypes to treat B-cell lymphomas have already been reported.[98,99]

Monoclonal Antibodies Made In Vitro

It must be remembered that monoclonal cold autoagglutinins that cause CHD were recognized as such[100] long before the technology was developed[89,90] to produce monoclonal antibodies in vitro. In CHD, of course, the production of a monoclonal antibody represents a malfunction of the individual's immune system. A few monoclonal antibodies (MoAbs) related to the Pr system have been made in vitro. The F11 MoAb of Ochiai et al[101] may well have anti-Pr_a specificity. In addition, other MoAbs that recognize NeuAc-containing epitopes in oligosaccharides attached to glycophorins A and B may be defining epitopes of the Pr antigens.[101-103] More often than not, mouse MoAbs directed against antigens carried on glycophorins A and B have had specificities against epitopes that include some of the protein backbone of the SGPs. Thus, as explained in detail in the section on biochemistry of the Pr antigens, these MoAbs define the MN system rather than Pr antigens. As will be seen, as far as the Pr determinants are concerned, the in vitro production of MoAbs has been more successful in the area of anti-idiotypes to Pr antibodies than in the production of MoAbs against the Pr antigens themselves.

Immune Red Cell Clearance

In concluding this section on the immunology of Pr antibodies, brief mention will be made of the mechanisms of red cell clearance used by the autoantibodies. Presumably, IgM anti-Pr cause CHD via complement-induced intravascular red cell hemolysis, with a smaller contribution through macrophage recognition of C3b-coated red cells, as with other IgM autoantibodies (for full details see reference 25). When the anti-Pr is IgG in nature, it seems that splenic sequestration and destruction of IgG-coated red cells (discussed in reference 25) occur.[36,38,39] As with other IgA antibodies, the mechanism of red cell clearance by IgA anti-Pr is not known. Such antibodies, including IgA anti-Pr, fail to activate complement[104] but no convincing case for the existence of tissue-bound macrophages capable of destroying IgA-coated red cells has yet been made. Recently, Salama et al[105] have suggested that some cold agglutinins are capable of direct, complement-independent hemolysis of red cells. The study included a number of IgM anti-I; 11 of 13 were reported to have caused some hemolysis. It is not yet known if this phenomenon occurs with antibodies other than anti-I, nor whether antibodies other than those that are IgM can effect such lysis.

Antigens Defined by Other Cold Agglutinins

In addition to the many Pr antigens, there are numerous others defined by cold-reactive autoagglutinins, some of which have been seen to cause CHD. As will become apparent, a number of these antigens share, with the Pr determinants, a dependence on NeuAc for structural integrity.

The Antigen Gd

The first two examples of anti-Gd were reported in 1977[106]; further examples have been found.[107-110] Some but not all of the known examples have caused CHD, most often of the type secondary to infection. As described below, the antigen defined was recognized as being glycolipid-dependent, hence choice of the name Gd. The Gd antigen is equally well-expressed on the red cells of adults (of the I and i phenotypes) and newborns. Protease-treated red cells retain Gd activity; the antigen is denatured when red cells are treated with neuraminidase.

One example of the antibody, anti-Gd(Kn), failed to react with ape and monkey red cells. A second example, anti-Gd(Hei), reacted strongly with those cells. Because of these findings and some made at the biochemical level, antibodies with the specificity of anti-Gd(Kn) are now called anti-Gd1; those with the specificity of anti-Gd(Hei) are called anti-Gd2.[111]

Konig et al[109] tested 192 sera containing anti-I for the concomitant presence of anti-Gd and anti-Fl. Three of the sera tested contained at least anti-I and anti-Gd. Since it has been shown[112-119] that the Gd (and Fl, see below) antigens are identical to structures identified as receptors for *M. pneumoniae*, Konig et al[109] concluded that the production of anti-Gd (and of anti-Fl) following infection with *M. pneumoniae* represents production of antibodies directed against those receptors. It will be noted that in many of the papers dealing with the *M. pneumoniae* receptor, the I and i antigens are named. In fact, the Gd (and Fl) structures represent I- and i-bearing structures to which terminal NeuAc has been added. It seems that the terminal NeuAc is an essential component in the receptor recognized by *M. pneumoniae*.[117]

Initial recognition of the fact that Gd is removed from red cells by treatment of those cells with neuraminidase, but that it is retained on protease-treated cells,[106,111] meant that while NeuAc must be essential for Gd antigen structure, the antigen must be carried on other than protease-sensitive glycoproteins of the red cell membrane. Indeed, it is now known[120] that glycophorins are Gd-inactive. Studies on glycolipids that include terminal NeuAc residues have shown[65,111,121-123] that Gd1 is represented by the immunodominant monosaccharide NeuAcα(2→3). While the monosaccharide is Gd1-active, alpha configuration is necessary. Gd2 is a little more complex in that the terminal NeuAc must be linked to galactose, ie, NeuAcα(2→3)Galβ1....

Such structures (Gd1 and Gd2) are present on many glycolipids of the red cell membrane, including those that carry I and i. Thus, as mentioned above, in some instances Gd1 and Gd2 are sialylated versions of I- and i-bearing chains. That the straight chain i structure is as suitable as the branched chain I structure (for details see reference 25) as a carrier for Gd is evidenced by the fact that I adult, i adult and i cord cells carry equally well developed Gd antigens. Indeed, this point has recently been proved at the biochemical level since Gd has been shown[124] to be present in linear and branched type 2 chains.

Findings that the antibody called anti-p[125-127] (also see Chapter 1) does not recognize the structure postulated to be a precursor of P, but recognizes sialylneolactotetrasylceramide (sialylosylparagloboside), a product of an alternative pathway,[128] that two of four anti-Gd showed enhanced reactions with Tj(a–) red cells[129] and that Tj(a–) red cells carry increased levels of the major Gd-active ganglioside,[129] suggest that anti-Gd would be a more appropriate name than anti-p for the antibody.[122]

The Antigen Sa

In 1980, Roelcke et al[120] gave the name anti-Sa to an IgM monoclonal cold agglutinin with kappa light chains that was causative of CHD. The Sa determinant was found to be present in about equal amounts on the red cells of adults of phenotypes I and i and those of newborns. Unlike I and i but similar to Pr and Gd, the Sa determinant was no longer detectable on red cells treated with neuraminidase. Unlike Pr, the Sa determinant was not completely denatured when red cells were treated with proteases. However, anti-Sa reacted less strongly with protease-treated than with untreated red cells and thus differed from anti-I and anti-i (whose reactions are enhanced) and anti-Gd (whose reactions are unchanged) when such cells are used.

These serologic findings suggested that Sa might be present on both protease-sensitive glycoproteins (copies of antigens removed by proteases) and protease-resistant glycolipids (copies of antigens resistant to proteases). Such suggestions were then confirmed at the biochemical level. Glycophorin A was shown[53,120] to be Sa-active and the structure NeuAcα(2→3)Gal was found to be immunodominant. The studies of Dahr et al[53] showed that the Sa determinants are included in oligosaccharides attached to the portion of glycophorin A that is fairly close to the red cell membrane. As discussed earlier, it is known[56] that in that region some of the side chains are trisaccharides (see Fig 4-1) and not the tetrasaccharides that occur as side chains near the NH_2 terminus of glycophorin A. Thus, it seems entirely possible that the Pr antigens are present in the tetra- and trisaccharides, while on membrane glycoproteins, Sa is predominantly located in the trisaccharides.

Unlike the Pr_1 and Pr_3 determinants that are confined to glycoproteins, Pr_2 and Sa are present on glycolipids as well.[65] On such components the immunodominant grouping of Sa seems to be NeuAcα(2→3)Galβ(1→4)Glc.[122] While Sa and Pr_2 are both optimally expressed on long chain gangliosides, Pr_2 is present on those of the neolacto and ganglio series, and Sa is restricted to the neolacto series.[65] Kundu et al[123] showed that the gangliosides that inhibited anti-Gd and anti-p (arguably the same antibody, see previous section) did not inhibit anti-Sa.

Pruzanski et al[130] used anti-Sa in cytotoxicity studies and found that it killed B cells from normal individuals somewhat more efficiently than it killed T cells from those donors. Anti-Sa was almost as active as anti-I and more active than anti-i in killing B cells from patients with chronic lymphocytic leukemia. T-helper cells from such patients were also highly susceptible to the actions of anti-Sa. Dorken et al[131] showed that similar to Gd but unlike Pr_1, the Sa determinant is not cell-type associated in patients with leukemia.

The Antigen Fl

In 1981, Roelcke[132] described a new specificity cold agglutinin, to which he gave the name anti-Fl, in the serum of a 69-year-old woman who had an immunoblastoma. Other examples of the antibody, which reacts with untreated and protease-treated red cells, have since been found.[109] The first example of anti-Fl reacted strongly (titer 2000) with I adult, weaker (titer 128) with i cord and weakest (titer <16) with i adult red cells. Thus, Fl was clearly different from Pr, Gd and Sa, which are present in about the same amounts on red cells of all three Ii phenotypes. Anti-Fl closely resembled anti-I in its initial reactions but was shown to differ from that antibody when it was found[132] to be nonreactive with neuraminidase-treated red cells.

As discussed in Chapter 2, NeuAc, which is specifically cleaved by neuraminidase, plays no role in the structure of any Ii blood group antigen. Biochemical characterization of the Fl determinant explained the serologic findings. The antigen is present in membrane glycoproteins and glycolipids that carry I[122,133]; its immunodominant carbohydrate is NeuAc.[122] In other words, Fl, as with Gd, can be thought of as being on an I-bearing structure to which terminal NeuAcα(2→3) has been added. Unlike Gd, which is formed by sialylation of straight chain (i-active) and branched chain (I-active) glycolipids so is present on I adult and i adult red cells, Fl is formed only by sialylation of the branched chain I-active structures. This, of course, explains exactly why anti-Fl closely resembles anti-I in its reactions with I adult, i adult and i cord cells.

Many glycolipids have been isolated from the red cell membrane. The one that carries the highest level of Fl has terminal NeuAcα(2→3) at the (1→3) branch and Fucα(1→2) at the (1→6) branch of the I-active branched structure.[134] The NeuAc residue is essential for Fl antigen integrity[65] and the Fuc(fucose) residue is necessary for optimal binding of anti-Fl.[134] Roelcke[135] reports that O_h (Bombay) red cells carry reduced levels of Fl. The close similarities between the I-active branched structures[136] and

Fl-active glycolipids[134] are thought[17] perhaps to account for the presence of both anti-I and anti-Fl in the sera of a number of patients.[109,137,138]

The Antigen Lud

In 1981, Roelcke[139] reported yet another cold agglutinin with a specificity different from any previously described. He named the new antibody anti-Lud. Similar to the Pr, Gd, Sa and Fl determinants but unlike those of the Ii blood group, Lud was denatured when red cells were treated with neuraminidase. Unlike the Pr antigens that are not detectable on protease-treated red cells, or Gd and Fl that are unaffected by such treatment, Lud is partially denatured by proteases and in that respect resembles Sa. Anti-Lud differs from anti-Sa in that it reacts less strongly with cord blood red cells than with those of adults. It differs from anti-Fl in that it reacts about equally with the red cells of adults of the I and i phenotypes. Thus, in terms of strongest to weakest reactions, anti-Lud places red cells in the order I adult and i adult > i cord, while anti-Fl places them in the sequence I adult > i cord > i adult. Anti-Sa, of course, reacts about equally with red cells of all three phenotypes.

If, as discussed, Gd is present on sialylated I- and i-bearing chains, Fl on sialylated I-bearing chains and Vo and Li (see next section) on sialylated i-bearing chains, it is tempting to speculate that Lud may represent a sialylated form of the structure that carries an antigen originally called I^T.[140-145] However, Pennington and Feizi[146] studied the agglutinating ability of type XIV pneumococcus antisera, which are somewhat similar to anti-Lud but do not require NeuAc in the structure(s) they recognize, and speculated that the antibodies might define a developmentally regulated increase of unsubstituted Type 1 chains.

Roelcke[17] suggests that the speculation could be taken one step further to propose that anti-Lud defines a structure on sialylated Type 1 chains. This, at first, seems to negate the suggestion of a possible relationship between Lud and I^T. If the original interpretation[140,141] of I^T as a "transitional" step in the development of I from i is correct, I^T should be present on Type 2, not Type 1 chains. However, there are data[142,143] that call into question such an interpretation. Thus, it seems possible that the antigen called I^T is actually carried on Type 1 chains and is not truly related to the I and i of Type 2 chains.

Kajii et al[147] reported a second example of anti-Lud, this one in a patient with chronic CHD. The antibody was IgM with kappa light chains and was used, as an eluate, in an immunoblotting procedure against red cell membranes separated by SDS-PAGE. The anti-Lud reacted with a protein of molecular weight of about 43 kDa. The requirement for NeuAc in the Lud determinant was confirmed when it was shown that anti-Lud failed to bind to membranes prepared from neuraminidase-treated red cells.

The Antigens Vo and Li

Anti-Vo, described in 1984 by Roelcke et al,[148] and anti-Li, described in 1985 by Roelcke,[149] both define protease-resistant, NeuAc-dependent antigens fully expressed only on i_{cord} and i_{adult} red cells. While both antibodies initially resemble anti-i in serologic studies, difference from that antibody is clear because both Vo and Li can be denatured by neuraminidase, while i cannot. Vo and Li differ in that treatment of intact red cells with neuraminidase denatures Li, while Vo is denatured by that enzyme only when the red cells have been previously treated with a protease. These findings led Roelcke[17] to suggest that Li is probably carried on sialylated neolacto chains of common length, while Vo is probably restricted to shorter versions of such chains.

The Antigen Defined by the Antibody IgM^{woo}

Kabat et al[150] described a human monoclonal IgM protein that complexed best with Galβ(1→3)GlcNAcβ(1→3)Galβ(1→4)Glc and that was specific for Galβ(1→3)GlcNAcβ(1→3)Gal. Readers with a better understanding than this author (that is not difficult to achieve) will recognize this as part of the Type 1 chain. The antibody, which recognized unsubstituted Type 1 chains, did not react with Type 2 chains that carry I and i. The antibody did not react with untreated or protease-treated human red cells but did react with such cells after they had been treated with neuraminidase. Picard et al[151] then showed that IgM^{woo} is specific for Type 1 chains but that its determinant on native chains is masked by NeuAc.[151] In this latter study a hybridoma-produced monoclonal antibody, FC10.2, with apparently the same specificity as IgM^{woo}, was used. As blood group serologists will know, treatment of human red cells with neuraminidase exposes the T receptor so that the cells become polyagglutinable.[25] That IgM^{woo} and FC10.2 were not anti-T was proved when it was shown that both complex with the structure Galβ(1→3)GlcNAcβ(1→3)Gal from Type 1 chains but not the structure Galβ(1→3)GalNAc, which is the T receptor.[151]

The Antigen Me

Salama et al[152] described an IgM cold agglutinin with kappa light chains that caused CHD in a patient with Waldenstrom's macroglobulinemia. The antibody was named anti-Me and it reacted equally well with the red cells of adults of the I phenotype and those of newborns. Since red cells of the i_{adult} phenotype were not available for testing, HEMPAS cells that are known[153,154] to have enhanced i were used. The HEMPAS cells reacted similarly to those from I adults and newborns. Anti-Me was shown to differ from the cold agglutinins that define I, i, Pr, Gd, Sa, Lud, Fl, Vo and Li in part because of its equal reactions with the red cells of adults and newborns and in part because its reactions were enhanced in tests against protease and neuraminidase-treated red cells.

Anti-Me was unusual in a number of other respects. First, it had a high thermal range and was apparently able to activate complement at temperatures up to 40 C. Second, it was hemolytic in vitro and caused hemolysis of I_{adult} and i_{cord} red cells over a wide range from pH 5.0 to pH 9.0. Third, tests with added human milk from eight different women were performed since it is known[155] that such milk inhibits some examples of anti-I (also see Chapter 2). Rather than causing inhibition, the addition of human milk markedly enhanced the reactivity of anti-Me. The enhancement was shown not to be due simply to presence of glucose or galactose in the milk. It was this last feature that resulted in selection of the name for the antigen; that is, Me for "milk enhanced."

The Antigen Om

Anti-Om[156] was an IgM cold agglutinin with kappa light chains from a 59-year-old man suffering from chronic CHD. It differed from the antibodies that define I, i, Fl, Vo and Li in that it reacted equally with red cells from adults of the I phenotype and with those of newborns. It differed from the antibodies that define Pr, Gd, Sa and Lud in that it gave enhanced reactions with protease and neuraminidase-treated red cells. In terms of previously recognized cold agglutinins, anti-Om was most similar to anti-Me. However, unlike anti-Me, anti-Om was markedly inhibited by human milk and by galactose. Thus, the antigen defined may be carried on a red cell membrane glycolipid and may include galactose, but not NeuAc, in its immunodominant configuration.

The Antigen Ju

In 1990, Gottsche et al[157] described a cold agglutinin in the serum of a 63-year-old man who had a 1-year history of mild CHD. The antibody was named anti-Ju after the patient and differed from the antibodies that define I, i, Fl, Vo and Li by reacting equally with red cells from adults and newborns. In titration studies, anti-Ju reacted equally with untreated, protease and neuraminidase-treated red cells at refrigerator temperatures. When the tests were done at 16 and 22 C, the antibody reacted best with untreated red cells, to lower titers with protease-treated and to its lowest titers with neuraminidase-treated red cells. Thus, Ju appeared to differ from Pr, Gd and Sa in being only partially denatured by neuraminidase. This conclusion was supported by the finding that neuraminidase-treated red cells were able, albeit slowly, to adsorb anti-Ju to exhaustion.

Human milk and sialyllactose did not inhibit anti-Ju. Thus, anti-Ju differed from anti-Om, which was inhibited by human milk. Its difference from anti-Me was based on the finding that anti-Me gives enhanced reactions with neuraminidase-treated red cells.

A Brief Summary of the Antigens Pr, Gd, Sa, Fl, Lud, Vo, Li, IgM^{woo}, Me, Om and Ju

The reactions of the cold agglutinins described in this chapter thus far, at first appear to represent a bewildering array of specificities. However, Roelcke[17] has pointed out that there are certain recognizable interrelations between many of them. The antibodies that define the Pr and Sa determinants appear to recognize epitopes, carried within O-glycans, that are dependent on the presence of NeuAc for immunogenic structure. They differ in that the Pr determinants appear to be present only in the O-glycans of glycoproteins while the Sa determinants appear to be present in the O-glycans of both glycoproteins and glycolipids. Possible exceptions are Pr_a, Pr^M and (the putative) Pr^N. Indeed, Dahr[67] has expressed reservations about the propriety of including determinants that may include contributions from the protein of glycophorins in their structure with the Pr antigens.

The Gd, Fl, Lud, Vo and Li determinants appear to be glycolipid-borne antigens. The I and i antigens are carried on lipid- and protein-linked branched and straight N-acetyl-lactosamine chains (see also Chapter 2). These Type 2 chains are the carrier molecules of ABH antigens; H specificity arises by fucosylation. An alternative substitution by sialylation may result in formation of the Gd, Fl, Vo and Li determinants. The specific sites (ie, I-bearing, i-bearing or both) of the NeuAc-dependent antigens are discussed in the sections describing those antigens.

The Lud and IgM^{woo} determinants may be present on Type 1 chains. Lud may be formed by the addition of NeuAc (sialylation) at specific sites on those chains. The determinant recognized by IgM^{woo} is known to be present but is apparently not accessible to its antibody until NeuAc is cleaved. Less can be said about the Me, Om and Ju antigens since little is known about them at the biochemical level. However, the determinants have some of the characteristics of glycolipid-borne antigens. The I and i determinants are found on both glycoproteins and glycolipids. While this chapter has stressed the probable glycolipid nature of the carriers of several of the other antigens, it should be borne in mind that future biochemical investigations may show the presence of small numbers of copies of some of those antigens on glycoproteins as well.

In an attempt to bring some order to this discussion, Table 4-3 presents some of the serologic characteristics of the antibodies described, Table 4-4 lists some minimum biochemical structures of the determinants defined and Table 4-5 shows possible sites of the antigens on red cells. It should

Table 4-3. Typical Reactions of Cold Agglutinins Other Than Anti-Pr*

Antibody Against	Test Red Cells			Prot	Nmdase	Notes About Antibodies and Antigens
	Adult I	Adult i	i cord			
Gd1	+	+	+	+	0	Nonreactive with ape and monkey red cells†
Gd2	+	+	+	+	0	Strongly reactive with ape and monkey red cells†
Sa	+	+	+	+→	0	Present on glycoproteins and glycolipids
Fl	+	+→→	+→	+	0	Possibly present on sialylated version of type 2, branched, I-bearing chains
Lud	+	+	+→	+→	0	May be present on sialylated type 1 chains
Vo	+→→	+	+	+	0	Antigen is denatured by neuraminidase only on red cells previously treated with a protease

					Comments
Li	+	+↓↓	+	+	0	Neuraminidase denatures antigen on untreated red cells
IgM^WOO‡	0	0	0		+	Antigen on type 1 chains, possibly blocked by NeuAc on untreated red cells
Me	+		+	+↑	+↑	Antibody reactivity enhanced by human milk
Om	+		+	+↑	+↑	Antibody inhibited by human milk and by galactose
Ju	+		+	+	+	Antibody not inhibited by milk. See text for effects of proteases and neuraminidase in tests at different temperatures

*Typical reactions are shown. For unusual reactions see text and references given therein
†May be present on branched, I-active and straight, i-active type 2 chains
‡Name refers to antibody; antigen defined has not been named

Prot = protease-treated adult I red cells, Nmdase = neuraminidase-treated adult I red cells, + = equal reactivity (in any horizontal line), +↓ = decreased reactivity, +↓↓ = reactivity decreased more than +↓, +↑ = reactivity enhanced, 0 = negative, blank spaces = no information

Table 4-4. Possible Minimal Structures of Some Determinants*

Gd1	NeuAcα(2→3). . . .
Gd2	NeuAcα(2→3)Galβ1. . . . (on glycoproteins)
Gd2	NeuAcα(2→3)Galβ(1→4)GlcNAc. . . . (on glycolipids)
Sa	NeuAcα(2→3)Galβ(1→4)Glc. . . . OR NeuAcα(2→3)Galβ(1→3)GalNAc. . . .
Fl	NeuAcα(2→3)Galβ(1→4)GlcNAcβ1 3 $Gal\beta$1. . . . 6 Fucα(1→2)Galβ(1→4)GlcNAcβ1
Lud†	NeuAcα(2→3)Galβ(1→3)GlcNAcβ1. . . .
Vo and Li†	NeuAcα(2→3)Galβ(1→4)GlcNAcβ(1→3). . . .
IgM^{woo}	Galβ(1→3)GlcNAc. . . . (see ‡)

*Minimal structures are shown. For additional structures required for optimal antibody binding and different linkage of minimal structures to glycoproteins and glycolipids, see text and references contained therein.
†Postulated minimal structures.
‡IgM^{woo} was shown not to bind to Galβ(1→3)GalNAc that is the T receptor.[151]
NeuAc = N-acetylneuraminic acid, Gal = D-galactose, Glc = D-glucose, GalNAc = N-acetyl-D-galactosamine, GlcNAc = N-acetyl-D-glucosamine, Fuc = L-fucose.

be remembered that the preparation of such tables perforce involves some oversimplification and use of the most usual characteristics. The text about each determinant and its antibody should be consulted for some differences that cannot be shown in tables.

The Antigen Rx

The last named antigen to be described in this chapter is defined by an antibody that has characteristics somewhat different from those already described. In 1980, Marsh et al[158] reported two examples of a complement-binding IgM autoagglutinin that reacted optimally at around 22 C. In one case the antibody clearly caused an acute but transient hemolytic episode; in the second case, in vivo destruction of red cells by the autoantibody seemed probable. The antibodies were unusual in two respects. First, they were more active over a temperature range of 12-22 C than at 4 C or 37 C.

Table 4-5. Major Characteristics and Possible Red Cell Membrane Sites of the Different Determinants

Pr: NeuAc-dependent, protease-sensitive. Carried in O-glycans (tetra- and trisaccharides) of at least glycophorins A and B. Pr_1 and Pr_3 are not present on glycolipids, for Pr_2 see text.

Sa: NeuAc-dependent, partially resistant to proteases. Carried in O-glycans (perhaps mainly in trisaccharides) of glycophorins A and B and glycolipids that probably do not carry I or i.

Gd: NeuAc-dependent, protease-resistant. Probably carried on Type 2 (glycolipid) chains of the branched (I-bearing) and linear (i-bearing) varieties.

Fl: NeuAc-dependent, protease-resistant. Probably carried on Type 2 (glycolipid) chains of the branched (I-bearing) variety but not on the linear (i-bearing) type. Fucose may be necessary for optimum binding of anti-Fl.

Lud: NeuAc-dependent, partially resistant to proteases. May be carried on Type 1 (glycolipid) chains that do not carry I or i. May possibly be related to I^T if that determinant is Type 1 chain-borne and not related to I and i, see text.

Vo and Li: NeuAc-dependent, protease-resistant. May be carried on Type 2 (glycolipid) chains of the linear (i-bearing) variety but not on the branched (I-bearing) type. The NeuAc residue involved in the Vo determinant may not be accessible to neuraminidase on native red cells.

IgM[woo]: NeuAc-independent. May be on Type 1 chains and blocked by NeuAc on native red cells.

Me: NeuAc-independent, protease-resistant. May be glycolipid-borne.

Om: NeuAc-independent, protease-resistant. May be glycolipid-borne and may include galactose in its immunodominant structure.

Ju: Partially but not wholly NeuAc-dependent. Partially protease-resistant, more so than to the actions of neuraminidase. May be glycolipid-borne with NeuAc contributing to tertiary structure (hence antibody binding) but not being essential for antigen integrity.

Second, the in vitro reactions of the antibodies were pH sensitive. Optimal reactions were seen in a saline system at pH6.5; as the pH was raised, the antibodies lost activity and were only very weakly reactive at pH8.0.

The antigen defined appeared to be present in about equal amounts on the red cells of adults of the I and i phenotypes; it was less well-developed on cord blood red cells. Unlike many other antigens described in this chapter, this one survived treatment of red cells with proteases and neuraminidase. In tests on 5000 samples from random donors, no nonreactive red cells were found. However, the antibodies were partially inhibited by human saliva and milk and were strongly inhibited by urine from humans with Sd(a+) red cells and by urine from guinea pigs. No inhibition was seen with urine from persons with Sd(a−) red cells. Thus, the antibody was clearly not anti-Sd^a (see Chapter 3) since it reacted equally (in titration) with Sd(a++) and Sd(a−) red cells, but appeared from the inhibition studies to have some sort of relationship to that antibody. Accordingly, the name anti-Sd^x was used.

After several other examples of this specificity had been studied (see below) the same group of investigators who first described the antibody showed[159] that it is not related to Sd^a at all. It was shown that in urine from Sd(a+) humans and from guinea pigs, there are charged molecules that had altered both the pH and salt concentration of the test system and had caused the antibody to become nonreactive. The urine from the Sd(a−) hospital patients had apparently not acted similarly. When urines from Sd(a+) persons were adjusted so that their conductivity was below the threshold at which nonspecific antibody inhibition occurred, they no longer had an inhibitory effect on the antibodies. In other words, inhibition of anti-Sd^x was not caused by presence of Sd^a on the T-H urinary glycoprotein (see Chapter 3) present in the urine of persons with Sd(a+) red cells.

The authors[159] renamed the antibody anti-Rx, after the first patient in whom it had been found. These observations illustrate that urine inhibition tests are not straightforward; the simple addition of urine to a sample can cause nonspecific inhibition of an antibody. A method suitable for the preparation of urine for use in inhibition studies has been published by Judd,[160] and is included in Chapter 5.

There is no doubt that anti-Rx (described by its original name of anti-Sd^x in the early publications) can be a clinically important antibody. Later, in 1980, Marsh et al[161] described four more cases of hemolytic anemia caused by the antibody; one of the patients died in an acute hemolytic episode. Among the first six patients in whom autoanti-Rx was found,[158,161] four had experienced a recent upper respiratory tract infection (URTI). Marsh et al[161] wondered if a cause-and-effect relationship existed between URTI and the production of anti-Rx. An incomplete IgG anti-Rx that caused "warm" antibody-induced hemolytic anemia was described by Denegri et al.[162]

Unnamed Antigens Defined by Cold Agglutinins

In spite of the exhaustive list of names of antigens defined by cold agglutinins, there are a number of reports of cases in which such antibodies caused severe hemolytic anemia but were not identified in terms of known specificities. In rare cases, hemolytic anemia is seen to be caused by both IgM and IgG and/or both cold- and warm-reactive autoantibodies in the patient.[144,163-169] Other papers give important information about CHD without necessarily naming the specificity of the causative autoantibody.[170-175] While all sera contain relatively weak, polyclonal cold agglutinins with restricted thermal range and anti-I specificity,[176,177] it is rare to find a high-titer cold agglutinin with a broad thermal range that is benign in vivo; one such antibody was described by Sniecinski et al.[178]

It is, of course, entirely possible that some of the unnamed cold agglutinins had one of the specificities described in this chapter but that the tests necessary for identification would have contributed nothing at the clinical level, so were not done. It is equally possible that some of them were studied before the specificities described herein were recognized and documented. A more sobering thought, which represents an equally plausible explanation, is that there remain new specificities, yet to be recognized and named.

References

1. Marsh WL, Jenkins WJ. Anti-Sp_1: The recognition of a new cold auto-antibody. Vox Sang 1968;15:177-86.
2. Roelcke D, Dorrow W. Besonderheiten der Reaktionsweise eines mit Plasmocytom-tA-Paraprotein identischen Kalteagglutinins. Klin Wochenschr 1968;46:126-31.
3. Bird GWG. Blood group antibody notation. Vox Sang 1969;17:468-9.
4. Roelcke D, Uhlenbruck G. Untitled letter to the Editor. Vox Sang 1970;18:478-9.
5. Marsh WL, Nichols ME. The effect of bacterial T-activating enzyme on the red cell Sp_1 antigen. Vox Sang 1969;17:217-20.
6. Roelcke D. A new serological specificity in cold antibodies of high titre: Anti-HD. Vox Sang 1969;16:76-9.
7. Roelcke D, Uhlenbruck G. Immunchemische Aspekte der Rezeptoren hochtitriger Kalteagglutinine. Z Immunforsch 1969; 137:333-42.
8. Roelcke D. Uhlenbruck G. Die unterschiedliche beeinflussung der Neuraminsaure-determinierten HD-rezeptoren durch behandlung humaner Erythrozyten mit verschiedenen Proteasen. Z Immunforsch 1969;138:273-82.

9. Roelcke D, Uhlenbruck G. Proteinase K: eine neue, serologisch anwendbare Pilz-protease. Z Med Mikrobiol Immunol 1969;155: 156-70.
10. Roelcke D, Uhlenbruck G, Bauer K. A heterogeneity of the HD receptor, demonstrable by HD-cold antibodies: HD_1/HD_2. Immunochemical aspects. Scand J Haematol 1969;6:280-7.
11. Roelcke D. Serological studies on the Pr_1/Pr_2 antigens using dog erythrocytes. Differentiation of Pr_2 from Pr_1 and detection of a Pr_1 heterogeneity: Pr_{1h}/Pr_{1d}. Vox Sang 1973;24:354-61.
12. Roelcke D, Ebert W, Geisen HP. Anti-Pr_3: Serological and immunochemical identification of a new anti-Pr subspecificity. Vox Sang 1976;30:122-33.
13. Roelcke D. Cold agglutination. Antibodies and antigens. Clin Immunol Immunopathol 1974;2:266-80.
14. Roelcke D, Ebert W, Anstee DJ. Demonstration of low titer anti-Pr cold agglutinins. Vox Sang 1974;27:429-44.
15. Geisen HP, Roelcke D, Rehn K, et al. Hochtitrige Kalteagglutinine der Spezifitat Anti-Pr nach Rotelninfektion. Klin Wochenschr 1975;53:767-72.
16. Roelcke D, Kreft H. Characterization of various anti-Pr agglutinins. Transfusion 1984;24:210-13.
17. Roelcke D. Cold agglutination. Transf Med Rev 1989;3:140-66.
18. Birgens HS, Dybkjaer E, Roelcke D. Identification of a cold agglutinin with anti-Pr_3 specificity. Scand J Haematol 1982;29:207-10.
19. Roelcke D, Forbes IJ, Zalewski PD, et al. A further subspecificity within human monoclonal anti-Pr cold agglutinins. Blut 1982;45: 109-14.
20. Romer W, Seelig HP, Lenhard V, Roelcke D. The distribution of I/i, Pr and Gd antigens in mammalian tissues. Invest Cell Pathol 1979; 2:157-62.
21. Roelcke D, Anstee DJ, Jungfer H, et al. IgG type cold agglutinins in children and corresponding antigens. Detection of a new Pr antigen: Pr_a. Vox Sang 1971;20:218-29.
22. Mollison PL. Blood transfusion in clinical medicine. 7th ed. Oxford: Blackwell Scientific Publications, 1983:322, 448.
23. Habibi B, Cregut R, Brossard Y, et al. Auto-anti-Pr_a: A "second" example in a newborn. Br J Haematol 1975;30:499-505.
24. Roelcke D, Dahr W, Kalden JR. A human monoclonal IgM kappa cold agglutinin recognizing oligosaccharides with immuno-dominant sialyl groups preferentially at the blood group M-specific peptide backbone of glycophorins: Anti-Pr^M. Vox Sang 1986;51: 207-11.
25. Issitt PD. Applied blood group serology. 3rd ed. Miami: Montgomery Scientific Publications, 1985.

26. Hinz CF Jr, Boyer JT. Dysgammaglobulinemia in the adult manifested as autoimmune hemolytic anemia. N Engl J Med 1963;269: 1329-35.
27. Feizi T. Lambda chains in cold agglutinins. Science 1976;156:1111-12.
28. Macris NT, Capra JD, Frankel GJ, et al. A lambda light chain cold agglutinin-cryomacroglobulin occurring in Waldenstrom's macroglobulinemia. Am J Med 1970;48:524-9.
29. Seligmann M, Brouet JC. Antibody activity of human myeloma globulins. Semin Hematol 1973;10:163-77.
30. Pruzanski W, Cowan DH, Parr DM. Clinical and immunochemical studies of IgM cold agglutinins with lambda type light chains. Clin Immunol Immunopathol 1974;2:234-45.
31. Isbister JP, Cooper DA, Blake HM, et al. Lymphoproliferative disease with IgM lambda monoclonal protein and autoimmune hemolytic anemia. Am J Med 1978;64:434-40.
32. Kuenn JW, Weber R, Teague PO, et al. Cryopathic gangrene with an IgM lambda cryoprecipitating cold agglutinin. Cancer 1978;42: 1826-33.
33. Lee CH, Cherian R, Hughes WG, et al. Lymphoproliferative disease with monoclonal IgM lambda gammopathy and cold agglutinin. Aust NZ J Med 1979;9:602-3.
34. Pascali E, Pezzoli A, Melato M, et al. Nodular lymphoma eventuating into lymphoblastic lymphoma with monoclonal IgM lambda cold agglutinin and Bence-Jones proteinuria. Acta Haematol 1980; 64:94-102.
35. Roelcke D. Unpublished data cited in Roelcke D. Cold agglutination. Transf Med Rev 1989;3:140-66.
36. Dellagi K, Brouet JC, Schenmetzler C, et al. Chronic hemolytic anemia due to a monoclonal IgG cold agglutinin with anti-Pr specificity. Blood 1981;57:189-91.
37. McGinnis MH, Wasniowska K, Dopf DA, et al. An erythrocyte Pr auto-antibody with sialoglycoprotein specificity in a patient with purine nucleoside phosphorylase deficiency. Transfusion 1985;25: 131-6.
38. Northoff H, Martin A, Roelcke D. An IgG kappa-monotypic anti-Pr_{1h} associated with fresh varicella infection. Eur J Haematol 1987;38: 85-8.
39. Curtis BR, Lamon J, Roelcke D, Chaplin H. Life threatening, antiglobulin test-negative, acute autoimmune hemolytic anemia due to a non-complement-activating IgG1 kappa cold antibody with Pr_a specificity. Transfusion 1990;30:838-43.
40. Angevine CD, Anderson BR, Barnett EV. A cold agglutinin of the IgA class. J Immunol 1966;96:578-86.

41. Garratty G, Petz LD, Brodsky I, et al. An IgA high-titer cold agglutinin with an unusual blood group specificity within the Pr complex. Vox Sang 1973;25:32-8.
42. Roelcke D. Specificity of IgA cold agglutinins: Anti-Pr_1. Eur J Immunol 1973;3:206-12.
43. Tonthat H, Rochant H, Henry A, et al. A new case of IgA kappa cold agglutinin with anti-Pr_{1d} specificity in a patient with persistent HB antigen cirrhosis. Vox Sang 1976;30:464-8.
44. Levine P, Celano MJ, Falkowski F. The specificity of the antibody in paroxysmal cold hemoglobinuria. Transfusion 1963;3:278-80.
45. Knapp T. The laboratory investigation of three cases of paroxysmal cold haemoglobinuria. Can J Med Technol 1964;26:172-6.
46. Wolach B, Heddle N, Barr RD, et al. Transient Donath-Landsteiner haemolytic anaemia. Br J Haematol 1981;48:425-34.
47. Judd WJ, Wilkinson SL, Issitt PD, et al. Donath-Landsteiner hemolytic anemia due to an anti-Pr-like biphasic hemolysin. Transfusion 1986;26:423-5.
48. Green ED, Curtis BR, Issitt PD, et al. Inhibition of an anti-Pr_{1d} cold agglutinin by citrate present in commercial red cell preservative solutions. Transfusion 1990;30:267-70.
49. Bell CA, Zwicker H, Spira S, Fischer ML. Transfusion in the presence of anti-Sp_1. Vox Sang 1973;25:271-80.
50. O'Neill P, Shulman IA, Simpson RB, et al. Two examples of low ionic strength-dependent autoagglutinins with anti-Pr_1 specificity. Vox Sang 1986;50:107-11.
51. Ebert W, Metz J, Weicker H, et al. Die Ficin-katalyscerte Fragmentierung von Erythrozytenmembran-glykoproteinen. Hoppe-Seyler's Z Physiol Chemie 1971;352:1309-18.
52. Roelcke D, Ebert W, Metz J, et al. I-, MN- and Pr_1/Pr_2-activity of human erythrocyte glycoprotein fractions obtained by ficin treatment. Vox Sang 1971;21:352-61.
53. Dahr W, Lichthardt D, Roelcke D. Studies on the receptor sites of the monoclonal anti-Pr and -Sa cold agglutinins. Prot Biol Fluids 1981;29:365-8.
54. Thomas DB, Winzler RJ. Structural studies on human erythrocyte glycoproteins. Alkali-labile oligosaccharides. J Biol Chem 1969;244:5943-6.
55. Adamany AM, Kathan RH. Isolation of a tetrasaccharide common to MM, NN and MN antigens. Biochem Biophys Res Comm 1969;37:171-8.
56. Lisowska E, Duk M, Dahr W. Comparison of alkali-labile oligosaccharide chains of M and N blood group glycopeptide from human erythrocyte membrane. Carbohydr Res 1980;79:103-13.
57. Dahr W. Unpublished observations cited in Roelcke D. Cold agglutination. Transf Med Rev 1989;3:140-66.

58. Ebert W, Fey J, Gartner CH, et al. Isolation and partial characterization of the Pr autoantigen determinants. Mol Immunol 1979;16: 413-19.
59. Garratty G, O'Neill P. Unpublished observations cited in O'Neill P, Shulman IA, Simpson RB, et al. Two examples of low ionic strength-dependent autoagglutinins with anti-Pr_1 specificity. Vox Sang 1986;50:107-11.
60. Suttajit M, Winzler RJ. Effect of modification of N-acetyl-neuraminic acid on the binding of glycoproteins of influenza virus and on susceptibility to cleavage by neuraminidase. J Biol Chem 1971;246: 3398-404.
61. Hoare DG, Koshland DE. A method for the quantitative modification and estimation of carboxylic acid groups in proteins. J Biol Chem 1967;242:2447-53.
62. Ebert W, Metz J, Roelcke D. Modifications of N-acetyl-neuraminic acid and their influence on the antigen activity of erythrocyte glycoproteins. Eur J Biochem 1972;27:470-2.
63. Lisowska E, Roelcke D. Differentiation of anti-Pr_1 and anti-Pr_2 sera with periodate-oxidized erythrocyte glycoproteins. Blut 1973;26: 339-41.
64. Tsai CM, Zopf DA, Wistar R Jr, et al. A human cold agglutinin which binds lacto-N-neotetraose. J Immunol 1976;117:717-20.
65. Uemura K, Roelcke D, Nagai Y, et al. The reactivities of human erythrocyte autoantibodies anti-Pr_2, anti-Gd, -Fl and -Sa with gangliosides in a chromatogram binding assay. Biochem J 1984;219: 865-74.
66. Anstee DJ. Blood group MNSs-active sialoglycoproteins of the human erythrocyte membrane. In: Sandler SG, Nusbacher J, Schanfield MS, eds. Immunobiology of the erythrocyte. New York: Alan R. Liss, 1980:67-98.
67. Dahr W. Immunochemistry of sialoglycoproteins in human red cell membranes. In: Vengelen-Tyler V, Judd WJ, eds. Recent advances in blood group biochemistry. Arlington VA: American Association of Blood Banks, 1986:23-65.
68. Tokunaga E, Sasakawa S, Tamaka K, et al. Two apparently healthy Japanese individuals of type M^kM^k have erythrocytes which lack both the blood group MN- and Ss-active sialoglycoproteins. J Immunogenet 1979;6:383-90.
69. Dahr W, Uhlenbruck G, Leikola J, et al. Studies on the membrane glycoprotein defect of En(a–) erythrocytes. 1. Biochemical aspects. J Immunogenet 1976;3:329-46.
70. Tanner MJA, Anstee DJ. The membrane change in En(a–) erythrocytes. Biochem J 1976;153:271-7.
71. Gahmberg CG, Myllylä G, Leikola J, Pirkola A. Absence of the major sialoglycoprotein in the membrane of human En(a–) erythrocytes

and increased glycosylation of band 3. J Biol Chem 1976;251:6108-16,
72. Issitt PD, Daniels G, Tippett P. Proposed new terminology for En^a (letter). Transfusion 1981;21:473-4.
73. Wilkinson SL, Issitt PD. Unpublished observations 1979 cited in Issitt PD. The MN blood group system. Cincinnati: Montgomery Scientific Publications, 1981:206.
74. Homberg JC, Krulik M, Habibi B, Debray J. Une agglutininé froid anti-Sp$_1$ au cours d'une leucémie lymphoide chroniqué complique de cirrhose hépatique. Nouv Rev Fr Hematol 1971;11:489-95.
75. Brunt DJ, Vengelen-Tyler V. Specificity studies of eight Pr antibodies (abstract). Transfusion 1981;21:615.
76. Dahr W, Uhlenbruck G, Issitt PD, Allen FH Jr. SDS-polyacrylamide gel electrophoretic analysis of the membrane glycoproteins from S–s–U– erythrocytes. J Immunogenet 1975;2:249-51.
77. Dahr W, Issitt P, Moulds J, Pavone B. Further studies on the membrane glycoprotein defects of S– s– and En(a–) erythrocytes. Hoppe-Seyler's Z Physiol Chemie 1978;359:1217-24.
78. Dahr W, Issitt PD, Uhlenbruck G. New concepts of the MNSs blood group system. In: Mohn JF, Plunkett RW, Cunningham RK, Lambert RM, eds. Human blood groups. Basel: Karger, 1977:197-205.
79. Rose VL, Kwaan HC. Anti-Pr cold hemagglutination associated with livedo reticularis. Am J Hematol 1985;19:419-21.
80. Silberstein LE, Robertson GA, Hannam Harris AC, et al. Etiologic aspects of cold agglutinin disease: Evidence for cytogenetically defined clones of lymphoid cells and the demonstration that an anti-Pr cold autoantibody is derived from a chromosomally aberrant B cell clone. Blood 1986;67:1705-9.
81. Pruzanski W, Roelcke D, Armstrong M, Manly MS. Pr and Gd antigens on human B and T lymphocytes and phagocytes. Clin Immunol Immunopathol 1980;15:631-41.
82. Ambrus M, Bajtai G. A case of IgG-type cold agglutinin disease. Haematologia 1969;3:225-35.
83. Roelcke D, Ebert W, Feizi T. Studies on the specificity of two IgM lambda cold agglutinins. Immunology 1974;27:879-86.
84. Ratkin GA, Osterland CK, Chaplin H Jr. IgG, IgA and IgM cold-reactive immunoglobulin in 19 patients with elevated cold agglutinins. J Lab Clin Med 1978;82:67-78.
85. Hsu TCS, Rosenfield RE, Burkart P, et al. Instrumented PVP-augmented antiglobulin tests. II. Evaluation of acquired hemolytic anemia. Vox Sang 1974;26:305-25.
86. Tschirhart D, Kunkel L, Shulman IA. Immune hemolytic anemia associated with biclonal cold autoagglutinins. Vox Sang 1990;59:222-6.

87. Feizi T, Kunkel HG, Roelcke D. Cross idiotypic specificity among cold agglutinins in relation to combining activity for blood group-related antigens. Clin Exp Immunol 1974;18:283-93.
88. Lecomte J, Feizi T. A common idiotype on human macroglobulins with anti-I and anti-i specificity. Clin Exp Immunol 1975;20:287-302.
89. Köhler G, Milstein C. Continuous cultures of fused cells secreting antibody of predefined specificity. Nature 1975;256:495-7.
90. Steinitz M, Klein G, Koskimies S, Makel O. EB virus-induced B lymphocyte cell lines producing specific antibody. Nature 1977; 269:420-2.
91. Evans SW, Feizi T, Childs R, Ling NR. Monoclonal antibody against a cross-reactive idiotypic determinant found on human autoantibodies with anti-I and -i specificities. Mol Immunol 1983;20:1127-31.
92. Stevenson FK, Wrightham M, Glennie MJ, et al. Antibodies to shared idiotypes as agents for analysis and therapy for human B cell tumors. Blood 1986;68:430-6.
93. Pfreundschuh M, Dorken B, Roelcke D, et al. Monoclonal anti-idiotype antibodies against lymphoma associated cold agglutinins. Blut 1983;46:111-14.
94. Romer W, Roelcke D, Rautenberg E. A new method for the preparation of anti-idiotypic antibodies against six different human cold agglutinins. Immunobiology 1983;164:380-9.
95. Jefferies LC, Stevenson FK, Goldman J, et al. Anti-idiotypic antibodies specific for a pathologic anti-Pr_2 cold agglutinin. Transfusion 1990;30:495-502.
96. Silberstein LE, Goldman J, Kant JA, Spitalnik SL. Comparative biochemical and genetic characterization of clonally related human B-cell lines secreting pathogenic anti-Pr_2 cold agglutinins. Arch Biochem Biophys 1988;264:244-52.
97. Thielemans K, Maloney DG, Meeker T, et al. Strategies for production of monoclonal anti-idiotype antibodies against human B cell lymphomas. J Immunol 1984;133:495-501.
98. Miller RA, Maloney DG, Warnke R, Levy R. Treatment of B-cell lymphoma with monoclonal anti-idiotypic antibody. N Engl J Med 1982;306:517-22.
99. Meeker TC, Lowder J, Maloney DG, et al. A clinical trial of anti-idiotype therapy for B cell malignancy. Blood 1985;65:1349-63.
100. Harboe M, van Furth R, Schubothe H, et al. Exclusive occurrence of kappa-chains in isolated cold haemagglutinins. Scand J Haematol 1965;2:259-66.
101. Ochiai Y, Furthmayr H, Marcus DM. Diverse specificities of five monoclonal antibodies reactive with glycophorin A of human erythrocytes. J Immunol 1983;131:864-8.

102. Anstee DJ, Edwards PAW. Monoclonal antibodies to human erythrocytes. Eur J Immunol 1982;12:228-32.
103. Anstee DJ. Contribution of monoclonal antibodies to the study of red cell membrane sialoglycoproteins. In: Cartron JP, Rouger P, Salmon C, eds. Red cell membrane glycoconjugates and related genetic markers. Paris: Librairie Arnette, 1983:37-42.
104. Romer W, Rother U, Roelcke D. Failure of IgA cold agglutinin to activate C. Immunobiology 1980;157:41-6.
105. Salama A, Gottsche B, Vaidya V, et al. Complement-independent lysis of human red blood cells by cold hemagglutinins. Vox Sang 1988;55:21-5.
106. Roelcke D, Riesen W, Geisen HP, Ebert W. Serological identification of the new cold agglutinin specificity anti-Gd. Vox Sang 1977;33:304-6.
107. Weber RJ, Clem LW. The molecular mechanism of cryoprecipitation and cold agglutination of an IgM lambda Waldenstrom's macroglobulin with anti-Gd specificity. Sedimentation analysis and localization of interacting sites. J Immunol 1981;127:300-5.
108. Staub CA. Cold reacting antibodies recognizing antigens dependent on N-acetylneuramic acid. Transfusion 1985;25:414-16.
109. Konig AL, Kreft H, Hengge U, et al. Coexisting anti-I and anti-Fl/Gd cold agglutinins in infections by *Mycoplasma pneumoniae*. Vox Sang 1988;55:176-80.
110. Pruzanski W, Roelcke D, Donnelly E, Lui L-C. Persisent cold agglutinins in AIDS and related disorders. Acta Haematol 1986;75:171-3.
111. Roelcke D, Brossmer R. Different fine specificities of human monoclonal anti-Gd cold agglutinins. Prot Biol Fluids 1984;31:1075-8.
112. Feizi T, Taylor-Robinson D, Shields MD, Carter RA. Production of cold agglutinins in rabbits immunized with human erythrocytes treated with *Mycoplasma pneumoniae*. Nature 1969;222:1253-6.
113. Costea N, Yakulis VJ, Heller P. Inhibition of cold agglutinins (anti-I) by *M. pneumoniae* antigens. Proc Soc Exp Biol Med 1972;139:476-9.
114. Lind K. Production of cold agglutinins in rabbits induced by *Mycoplasma pneumoniae*, *Listeria monocytogenes* or *Streptococcus MG*. Acta Pathol Microbiol Immunol Scand [B] 1973;81:487-96.
115. Feizi T. The monoclonal antibodies of cold agglutinin syndrome. Immunochemistry and biochemical aspects of their target antigens with special reference to the Ii antigens. Med Biol 1980;58:123-7.
116. Tardieu M, Epstein RL, Weiner HL. Interaction of viruses with cell surface receptors. Int Rev Cytol 1982;80:27-61.
117. Loomes LM, Uemura K, Childs RA, et al. Erythrocyte receptors for *Mycoplasma pneumoniae* are sialylated oligosaccharides of Ii antigen type. Nature 1984;307:560-3.
118. Feizi T, Gooi HC, Loomes LM, et al. Cryptic I antigen activity and *Mycoplasma pneumoniae*-receptor activity associated with sialo-

glycoprotein GP-2 of bovine erythrocyte membranes. Biosci Rep 1984;4:743-9.
119. Loomes LM, Uemura K, Feizi T. Interaction of *Mycoplasma pneumoniae* with erythrocyte glycolipids of I and i antigen types. Infect Immun 1985;47:15-20.
120. Roelcke D, Pruzanski W, Ebert W, et al. A new human monoclonal cold agglutinin Sa recognizing terminal N-acetyl-neuraminyl groups on the cell surface. Blood 1980;55:677-81.
121. Roelcke D, Brossmer R, Riesen W. Inhibition of human anti-Gd cold agglutinins by siallylactose. Scand J Immunol 1978;8:179 85.
122. Roelcke D, Brossmer R, Ebert W. Anti-Pr, -Gd and related cold agglutinins. Human monoclonal antibodies against neuraminyl groups. Prot Biol Fluids 1981;29:619-22.
123. Kundu SK, Marcus DM, Roelcke D. Glycosphingolipid receptors for anti-Gd and anti-p cold agglutinins. Immunol Lett 1982;4:263-7.
124. Roelcke D, Hengge U, Kirschfink M. Neolacto (type-2 chain)-sialoautoantigens recognized by human cold agglutinins. Vox Sang 1990;59:235-9.
125. Engelfriet CP, Beckers D, von dem Borne AEGKr, et al. Haemolysins probably recognizing the antigen p. Vox Sang 1972;23:176-81.
126. Metaxas MN, Metaxas-Buhler M, Tippett P. A "new" antibody in the P blood group system (abstract). Book of Abstracts, 14th Congress of the International Society of Blood Transfusion (Helsinki). Paris: ISBT, 1975:95.
127. Issitt CH, Duckett JB, Osborne BM, et al. Another example of an antibody reacting optimally with p red cells. Br J Haematol 1976; 34:19-23.
128. Schwarting GA, Marcus DM, Metaxas M. Identification of sialosylparagloboside as the erythrocyte receptor for an "anti-p" antibody. Vox Sang 1977;32:257-61.
129. Roelcke D. Reaction of anti-Gd, anti-Fl and anti-Sa cold agglutinins with p erythrocytes. Vox Sang 1984;46:161-4.
130. Pruzanski W, Armstrong M, Roelcke D. New antigenic determinant (Sa) on human lymphocytes and phagocytes. Blut 1981;43:307-13.
131. Dorken B, Roelcke D, Bohn B, Hunstein W. Analysis of carbohydrate determinants on membranes of leukemic leucocytes using naturally-occurring monoclonal human antibodies (cold agglutinins). Prot Biol Fluids 1981;29:623-6.
132. Roelcke D. A further cold agglutinin, Fl, recognizing a N-acetylneuraminic acid determined antigen. Vox Sang 1981;41:98-101.
133. Ebert W, Roelcke D, Weicker H. The I antigen of human red cell membrane. Eur J Biochem 1975;53:505-15.
134. Kannagi R, Roelcke D, Peterson KA, et al. Characterization of an epitope (determinant) structure in a developmentally regulated glycolipid antigen defined by a cold agglutinin Fl, recognition of

alpha-sialosyl and alpha-L-fucosyl groups in a branched structure. Carbohydr Res 1983;120:143-57.
135. Roelcke D. Unpublished observations 1988, cited in Roelcke D. Cold agglutination. Transf Med Rev 1989;3:140-66.
136. Feizi T, Childs RA, Watanabe K, Hakomori S. Three types of blood group I specificity among monoclonal anti-I auto-antibodies revealed by analogues of a branched erythrocyte glycolipid. J Exp Med 1979;149:975-80.
137. Konig AL, Kather H, Roelcke D. Autoimmune hemolytic anemia by coexisting anti-I and anti-Fl cold agglutinins. Blut 1984;49:363-8.
138. Roelcke D, Weber MT. Simultaneous occurrence of anti-Fl and anti-I cold agglutinins in a patient's serum. Vox Sang 1984;47:122-4.
139. Roelcke D. The Lud cold agglutinin: A further antibody recognizing N-acetylneuraminic acid-determined antigens not fully expressed at birth. Vox Sang 1981;41:316-18.
140. Booth PB, Jenkins WJ, Marsh WL. Anti-I^T. A new antibody of the I blood group system occurring in certain Melanesian sera. Br J Haematol 1966;12:341-4.
141. Booth PB. The occurrence of weak I^T red cell antigen among Melanesians. Vox Sang 1972;22:64-72.
142. Garratty G, Hafleigh B, Dalziel J, Petz LD. An IgG anti-I^T detected in a Caucasian American. Transfusion 1972;12:325-9.
143. Garratty G, Petz LD, Wallerstein RD, Fudenberg HH. Autoimmune hemolytic anemia in Hodgkin's disease associated with anti-I^T. Transfusion 1974;14:226-31.
144. Freedman J, Newlands M, Johnson CA. Warm IgM anti-I^T causing autoimmune hemolytic anaemia. Vox Sang 1977;32:135-42.
145. Hafleigh EB, Wells RF, Grumet FC. Nonhemolytic IgG anti-I^T. Transfusion 1978;18:592-7.
146. Pennington J, Feizi T. Horse anti-type 14 pneumococcus sera behave as cold agglutinins recognizing developmentally regulated antigens apart from the Ii antigens on human erythrocytes. Vox Sang 1982;43:253-8.
147. Kajii E, Ikemoto S, Miura Y. Localization of the Lud antigen by immunoblotting (letter). Vox Sang 1988;54:248.
148. Roelcke D, Kreft H, Pfister AM. Cold agglutinin Vo. An IgM lambda monoclonal human antibody recognizing a sialic acid determined antigen fully expressed on newborn erythrocytes. Vox Sang 1984;47:236-41.
149. Roelcke D. Li cold agglutinin: A further antibody recognizing sialic acid-dependent antigens fully expressed on newborn erythrocytes. Vox Sang 1985;48:181-3.
150. Kabat EA, Liao J, Shyong J, et al. A monoclonal IgM lambda macroglobulin with specificity for lacto-N-tetraose in a patient with bronchogenic carcinoma. J Immunol 1982;128:540-4.

151. Picard JK, Loveday D, Feizi T. Evidence for sialylated type 1 blood group chains on human erythrocyte membranes revealed by agglutination of neuraminidase-treated erythrocytes with Waldenstrom's macroglobulin IgM^{woo} and hybridoma antibody FC10. Vox Sang 1985;48:26-33.
152. Salama A, Pralle H, Mueller-Eckhardt C. A new red blood cell cold autoantibody (anti-Me). Vox Sang 1985;49:277-84.
153. Crookston JH, Crookston MC, Burnie KL, et al. Hereditary erythroblastic multinuclearity associated with a positive acidified-serum test: A type of congenital dyserythropoietic anemia. Br J Haematol 1969;17:11-20.
154. Crookston JH, Crookston MC. HEMPAS: Clinical, hematological and serological features. In: Salmon C, ed. Blood groups and other red cell surface markers in health and disease. New York: Masson Publishing, 1982:29-38.
155. Marsh WL, Nichols ME, Allen FH Jr. Inhibition of anti-I sera by human milk. Vox Sang 1970;18:149-54.
156. Kajii E, Ikemoto S. A cold agglutinin: Om. Vox Sang 1989;56:104-6.
157. Gottsche B, Salama A, Mueller-Eckhardt C. Autoimmune hemolytic anemia caused by a cold agglutinin with a new specificity (anti-Ju). Transfusion 1990;30:261-2.
158. Marsh WL, Johnson CL, Øyen R, et al. Anti-Sd^x: A "new" auto-agglutinin related to the Sd^a blood group. Transfusion 1980;20:1-8.
159. Bass LS, Rao AH, Goldstein J, Marsh WL. The Sd^x-antigen and antibody: Biochemical studies on the inhibitory property of human urine. Vox Sang 1983;44:191-6.
160. Judd WJ. Methods in immunohematology. Miami: Montgomery Scientific Publications, 1988:230.
161. Marsh WL, Johnson CL, DiNapoli J, et al. Immune hemolytic anemia caused by auto-anti-Sd^x: A report on six cases (abstract). Transfusion 1980;20:647.
162. Denegri JF, Nanji AA, Sinclair M, et al. Autoimmune hemolytic anemia due to immunoglobulin G with anti-Sd^x specificity. Acta Haematol 1983;69:19-22.
163. Moore JA, Chaplin H Jr. Autoimmune hemolytic anemia associated with an IgG cold incomplete antibody. Vox Sang 1973;24:236-45.
164. Crookston JH. Hemolytic anemia with IgG and IgM autoantibodies and alloantibodies. Arch Intern Med 1975;135:1314-5.
165. Freedman J, Newlands M. Autoimmune haemolytic anaemia with the unusual combination of both IgM and IgG autoantibodies. Vox Sang 1977;32:61-8.
166. Sokol RJ, Hewitt S, Stamps BK. Autoimmune haemolysis: An 18-year study of 865 cases referred to a regional transfusion centre. Br Med J 1981;1:2023-7.
167. Sokol RJ, Hewitt S, Stamps BK. Autoimmune hemolysis: Mixed warm and cold type antibody. Acta Haematol 1983;69:266-74.

168. Shulman IA, Branch DR, Nelson JM, et al. Autoimmune hemolytic anemia with both cold and warm autoantibodies. J Am Med Assoc 1985;253:1746-8.
169. Silberstein LE, Shoenfeld Y, Schwartz RS, et al. A combination of IgG and IgM autoantibodies in chronic cold agglutinin disease: Immunologic studies and response to splenectomy. Vox Sang 1985; 48:105-9.
170. Wortman J, Rosse W, Logue G. Cold agglutinin autoimmune hemolytic anemia in nonhematologic malignancies. Am J Hematol 1979; 6:275-83.
171. Crisp D, Pruzanski W. B-cell neoplasms with homogeneous cold-reacting antibodies (cold agglutinins). Am J Med 1982;72:915-22.
172. Pruzanski W, Katz A. Cold agglutinins—antibodies with biological diversity. Clin Immunol Rev 1984;3:131-68.
173. Sandhaus LM, Raska K, Wu HV. Diffuse large-cell lymphoma with monoclonal IgM kappa and cold agglutinin. Am J Clin Pathol 1986;86:120-3.
174. Silberstein LE, Berkman EM, Schreiber AD. Cold hemagglutinin disease associated with IgG cold reactive antibody. Ann Intern Med 1987;106:238-42.
175. Pruzanski W, Jacobs H, Saito S, et al. Cryptic cold agglutinin activity of monoclonal macroglobulins. Am J Hematol 1987;26:167-74.
176. Jackson VA, Issitt PD, Francis BJ, et al. The simultaneous presence of anti-I and anti-i in sera. Vox Sang 1968;15:133-41.
177. Issitt PD, Jackson VA. Useful modifications and variations of technics in work on I system antibodies. Vox Sang 1968;15:152-3.
178. Sniecinski I, Margolin K, Shulman I, et al. High-titer, high-thermal-amplitude cold autoagglutinin not associated with hemolytic anemia. Vox Sang 1988;55:26-29.

In: Moulds JM and Woods LL, eds.
Blood Groups: P, I, Sd^a and Pr
Arlington, VA: American Association of Blood Banks, 1991

5

Serology of P, I, Sd^a, Rx and Pr

Marilyn K. Moulds, MT(ASCP)SBB

P, I, Sd^a, Rx and Pr collectively are a group of red blood cell (RBC) membrane antigens recognized by cold agglutinins. The antigens are also widely distributed in tissues and biologic fluids. Human antibodies directed at antigens in the P and I blood groups have been both allo- and autoantibodies. Anti-Sd^a has only been described as an alloantibody. The Rx and Pr cold agglutinins are autoantibodies.

Detection of these cold agglutinins in routine serologic testing is important when they are considered to be pathologic—ie, implicated in hemolytic transfusion reactions, hemolytic disease of the newborn, cold agglutinin disease, autoimmune hemolytic anemia or associated with viral infections. Identifying the exact antibody specificities and distinguishing between allo- and autoantibody can assist in determining whether the antibodies have the potential to be clinically significant and in some cases can aid in clinical diagnosis and treatment of patients.

P

Antigens

The P_1 and P_2 phenotypes are recognized in the majority of individuals, with P_1k, P_2k and p being exceptional or rare.

One can distinguish strong, normal and weak P_1 phenotypes, which often creates problems in testing RBCs for the antigen and in identifying the antibody. The P1 antigen is frequently poorly developed at birth.

Luke (LKE) is an antigen not present on the RBCs of the rare phenotypes p and P^k and 2% of random donors. Initially, it was thought that weakly positive or negative reactors were seen more frequently with P_2

Marilyn K. Moulds, MT(ASCP)SBB, Director, Consultation and Education, Gamma Biologicals, Inc, Houston, Texas than P_1 RBCs and with A_1 and A_1B RBCs than with O, A_2, A_2B and B RBCs.[1] Recent studies with a monoclonal antibody (see Monoclonal section below) have not totally supported these data.[2]

IP, IP_1, I^TP_1 and iP_1 are antigens relating P and P1 to I or i.

Antibodies

Human

Alloanti-P1 occurs frequently in sera of P_2 individuals as a naturally occurring antibody. It is usually a cold-reactive IgM antibody with little clinical importance. However, due to variation in strength of P1 antigen from person to person, anti-P1 can be difficult to identify if routine antibody resolution techniques do not include a room temperature phase of testing or potentiators of agglutination (enzymes) that will detect the weak P_1 phenotype. Also, if anti-P1 occurs in combination with other allo- and/or autoantibodies, it may be difficult to elucidate its specificity and/or specificity of other accompanying alloantibodies that are clinically significant. The discovery that human and sheep hydatid cyst fluid (HCF)—if scolices are present[3]—and pigeon egg whites[4] contain P1 substance that will inhibit activity of anti-P1 has helped greatly in serologic investigation of this antibody (technique will be discussed under Inhibition). It is interesting to note that anti-P1 has been detected in high titer in sera of P_2 individuals who are pigeon breeders[5] or infested with hydatid cysts[3,6] or hepatic distomiasis.[6,7]

A case of alloanti-P1 in a P1+ person has been reported.[8] Unfortunately, the patient died and sufficient studies before or after his illness were not possible to explain the exact nature of the antibody. His P1 typing was weak to moderate. The antibody was also very weak. The patient was an active pigeon breeder for many years.

Alloanti-P in P_1k and P_2k individuals as well as alloanti-PP_1P^k produced by p persons are naturally occurring, often of high titer, active at 37 C and can show hemolysis in vitro (especially with enzyme pretreated RBCs). Fortunately, these phenotypes are rare since antibodies produced by these individuals have the potential for being clinically significant (especially if they are hemolytic in vitro). Anti-P is not inhibited with HCF but anti-P^k (part of anti-PP_1P^k) is.

Anti-Luke (anti-LKE) was found in the serum of a patient with Hodgkin's disease.[9] The antibody did not react with rare p and P^k RBCs and 2% of P+ people. Only four human examples of the antibody have been described,[10] and studies with the first three examples of the antibody did not give conclusive results to establish the relationship of Luke to P. The family study on the patient with the fourth human example of anti-LKE confirmed that P^k expression is greater on cells of LKE− members than LKE+ members. Expression of LKE varied in this family depending on P1 phenotype.[10(p237)] Recent testing with the human antibodies and a monoclonal antibody has also given us a better understanding of association of Luke to P.[2(pp87-91)]

Autoanti-P_1PP^k was reported by Vos[11] in the sera of one-third of Australian women threatened by a second miscarriage, as a transient antibody that hemolyzed their own RBCs in vitro but not in vivo. They were of the P_1 or P_2 phenotype.

The Donath-Landsteiner antibody in paroxysmal cold hemoglobinuria (PCH), first described in 1904,[12] is unique in that it is biphasic. Biphasic hemolysins are antibodies that agglutinate RBCs at low temperatures and hemolyze RBCs after incubation at 4 C followed by incubation at 37 C. Almost all workers agree that complement is essential for hemolysis to occur in the warm phase, but all are not in agreement as to the need for complement in the cold phase.[13]

In 1965 Worlledge and Russo[14] studied sera of 11 patients with PCH, and serologic tests revealed that:

1. Antibody specificity is very close to alloanti-P produced by rare P^k individuals.
2. The antibody is not enhanced when tested with enzyme pretreated RBCs, as would be an anti-P1.
3. Pig HCF, at a dilution of 1 in 40, does not inhibit the antibody but usually inhibits anti-P1.

The anti-P biphasic antibody in PCH would rarely cause crossmatching difficulties, and patients usually do not require transfusions. Recognition of presence of this unusual biphasic antibody in a patient's serum could assist in differential diagnosis of PCH from immune hemolysis. A recent report describes a serum containing both IgM bithermic anti-P and cold anti-I^T.[15] The serum gave a Donath-Landsteiner-like reaction and contained a cold agglutinin strongest with cord RBCs, then I adult RBCs and weakest with ii adult RBCs (anti-I^T). These antibodies were associated with fatal autoimmune hemolytic anemia. Thus, it is important that all blood group serologists be familiar with the Donath-Landsteiner test. Appendix 5-1 outlines the procedure.[16,17]

Engelfriet and coworkers in 1972 described a serum containing biphasic hemolysins and warm hemolysins with anti-p specificity.[18] The serum first contained biphasic hemolysins reactive with adult P_1 or P_2 RBCs but gave stronger reactions with pp RBCs. A second serum sample appeared to contain pure anti-p. In 1975 Issitt et al,[19] described a second example of anti-p. Interestingly, nine of 19 cord blood samples were reactive (all nine were P_2).

Anti-IP,[20] -IP_1,[21] -I^TP_1[22] and -iP_1[23] are autoantibodies directed against antigenic determinants produced by actions of P and/or P^1 and I genes. Although uncommon, the specificities of these antibodies can be difficult to elucidate, for the P1 component of the antibody would be inhibited with HCF or pigeon egg white but the I and/or i components may or may not be inhibited.

In 1974 Judd[24] reported on an autoantibody that was pH-dependent and had P specificity. It was reactive only below pH 6.0. The antibody was detected because EDTA (ethylenediaminetetraacetic acid, dipotassium salt) was present in the saline solution used in automated ABO and D typing of donor blood samples. The pH of the reaction medium is 5.5.

Two examples of LISS (low ionic strength saline) dependent autoantibodies with apparent anti-P specificity were reported in 1982.[25] One antibody was only reactive in LISS solution at room temperature (RT). The second was reactive in LISS solution at RT, 37 C and by an IAT. In a letter to the editor, Cohen and Nelson[26] reported on an autoanti-P reactive only in LISS solution in a patient with hemolysis. They suggested that the anti-P could have been associated with in vivo hemolysis, since the bilirubin levels decreased after the anti-P disappeared. The anti-P was only reactive by LISS techniques at room temperature.

Monoclonal

Monoclonal anti-P and -P^k have been identified.[2(pp86-7)] Two mouse monoclonal antibodies, MC813-70 and MC631, were found that did not react with p and P^k RBCs. However, one (MC813-70) did not react with LKE–RBCs and one (MC631) did. The monoclonal anti-P^k demonstrated that P_1LKE– RBCs gave stronger reactions than P_1LKE+ RBCs. Also, it was confirmed that P+LKE– persons have a stronger P^k antigen than P+LKE+ persons.

Tippett and Wilfert[27] evaluated reactivity of a monoclonal antibody MAB077, an anti-P1. At 4 C this antibody did not agglutinate RBCs with weak P1 antigens. If papain-treated RBCs were tested, all P1+ samples reacted. Papain was most effective in enhancing reactions with MAB 077, with pronase next, then α-chymotrypsin and lastly trypsin-sialidase. Papain-treated cord RBCs (9 of 10) were reactive with MAB077, but only 3 of 10 were reactive with polyclonal anti-P1. Thus, MAB077 might be a useful reagent for P1 phenotyping cord RBCs, but only if the RBCs were first treated with papain.

These workers also investigated reactivity of MAB078, an anti-P^k. Papain-treated P_1k, P_2k and P_1LKE– RBCs were agglutinated at 21 C and 4 C, but P_2LKE– RBCs were agglutinated at 4 C but not 21 C. This antibody showed that P^k expression on P_1LKE– RBCs is greater than that on P_2LKE– RBCs.

It is obvious that monoclonal antibodies can be useful reagents but may require careful standardization of techniques if used for routine phenotyping. Monoclonal antibodies directed at antigens in the P and I blood groups may also show the same variation in specificities seen with human antibodies—ie, reactivity dependent on ABO, H and/or Lewis antigens on RBCs tested.

Inhibition

Anti-P1 and -P^k can be inhibited with P1 substance obtained from hydatid cysts containing scolices, turtle dove egg white, and synthetic oligosaccharide, glucose, or galactose haptens covalently bound to crystalline silicate particles. The latter P1 substance technique will not be outlined here but can be found in the paper by Cowles and Blumberg.[28] Appendix 5-2 outlines the procedure for inhibition of anti-P1 with HCF and/or avian (pigeon) egg white.[29,30(pp118-20)]

Marsh and Øyen[31] cautioned that before fluid from hydatid cysts is used for inhibition, it must be sterilized by filtration, as the hooklets of the parasite are highly infectious. The fluid is also alkaline (pH 8.4), and a buffer solution must be added to adjust the pH to 7.0.

I

Antigens

I and i antigens do not belong to a discrete blood group system but are grouped as a collection (ISBT #207). They are defined by autologous human antibodies. There is a great difference in reactivity and number of sites between adult and cord RBCs. The first year after birth the i reactivity decreases and the maximum level of I reactivity is reached after 2 years. Classic I and i phenotypes are I, I intermediate, i cord, i_1 and i_2.

Almost all individuals have i antigen, and RBCs of the very rare I– adult individuals may react weakly with some examples of anti-I.[1(pp177-8)] There is a slight increase in number of I sites on Bombay (O_h) RBCs. The i antigen is depressed on RBCs of Lu(a–b–) individuals of the dominant type. Depressed I with enhanced i reactivity has been described on RBCs of leukemia and preleukemia patients, in myeloproliferative syndromes, bone marrow aplasia, paroxysmal nocturnal hemoglobinuria, acquired hemolytic anemia and dyserythropoiesis. In some diseases, I antigen can also be enhanced when i is not. Enhanced i has been observed in repeated phlebotomy, acanthocytosis, sideroblastic anemia, megaloblastic anemia, in HEMPAS RBCs[1(p187)] and congenital hypoplastic anemia (Blackfan-Diamond syndrome).[32,33]

Enhanced and/or depressed reactivity of I and/or i in the above conditions can influence serologic test results during investigation of patient sera containing cold agglutinins. For example, if the I antigen is suppressed, an autoantibody could appear to be alloantibody. The patient's autoanti-I would not react well or would not react at all with autologous RBCs.

Antibodies

Anti-I

Alloanti-I is rare, since RBCs of only one in 10,000 individuals lack I antigen. The antibody is usually IgM and of low titer. Most I– adult individuals have been detected by deliberate search using anti-I to screen donor RBCs. The RBCs of these individuals type strongly i+, although the I–i– phenotype has been reported in India.

If a patient appears to have alloanti-I in the serum (ie, autologous RBCs do not react), the patient's RBCs should be typed for both I and i. However, it is very important to know the diagnosis of the patient to eliminate the possibility of depressed reactivity of both I and i due to association with disease. Enzyme pretreated RBCs bind cold agglutinins with a much higher affinity than untreated RBCs. The patient's enzyme pretreated RBCs should be tested with the serum and with different examples of anti-I (using appropriate controls). Autoanti-I can be detected as a naturally occurring IgM antibody in the sera of all adults, if a deliberate search is made. With recent streamlining of antibody detection techniques (elimination of room temperature phase of testing) and routine use of IgG antiglobulin serum, fewer problems are seen due to this cold agglutinin.

The use of some commercial LISS additives containing potentiators of agglutination (low ionic/high molecular additive solution) will, of course, enhance reactivity of autoanti-I (especially in the immediate-spin phase of testing and sometimes in the 37 C phase). If the presence of a cold agglutinin is suspected, a LISS reagent (low ionic strength additive solution) without potentiators could be used.

In 1984, Reviron et al[34] reported a case of autoanti-I enhanced in the presence of sodium azide. This led to difficulty in determining the ABO blood group of the patient using unwashed RBCs.

Examples of "pure" autoanti-I are generally detected in sera of group O individuals. The antibody observed in sera of group A, B and AB persons usually has IH(HI) specificity. From a practical or serologic standpoint, group O screening RBCs will often be reactive with a patient's serum, while crossmatches with ABO-specific donor units will be compatible. This is by far the most frequently encountered cold agglutinin problem in the blood bank. Bird and Wingham[35] first published in 1977 a report of an erythrocyte autoagglutinin with the unusual specificity of Hi. No additional examples were reported until 1990 when Pierce[36] and coworkers described three further examples. Group O cord RBCs were reactive to the same strength as group O adult RBCs. Group A_2 cord RBCs were less reactive than group O adult and cord RBCs, and group A_1 cord RBCs were even weaker in reactivity or nonreactive. This unusual specificity would only be suspected if group O cord RBCs were used routinely in antibody resolution techniques.

Anti-I^T

Anti-I^T is an uncommon antibody reported in isolated populations in Melanesia, Venezuela and North America. Anti-I^T (transition) reacts strongly with cord RBCs, weakly with adult RBCs and even more weakly with i adult RBCs. In 1975, Dzierzkowa-Borodej et al[37] evaluated 12 anti-I sera and classified these into various specificities: I^F (fetal), I^D (developed) and I^S (secreted). Some sera contained combinations of two or more kinds of specificities (ie, anti-I^D + -I^F, anti-I^D + -i, anti-I^D + -I^S and anti-I^D + -I^F + -I^S). These components of I were established by comparing agglutination with untreated and neuraminidase-treated adult and cord RBCs. Anti-IA, -IB and -IHLe^{bH} specificities have been classified based on serologic reactivity with RBCs of differing I, ABO and Lewis phenotypes.

Anti-i

Anti-i is rarely seen in sera of "normal" individuals. The antibody reacts preferentially with cord RBCs (i) compared to adult (I) RBCs. It is occasionally seen in lymphoproliferative disorders and other disease states, and Horowitz and workers[38] showed that anti-i is frequently encountered in sera of patients (31.8% of cases) with heterophile-antibody-positive Epstein-Barr virus (EBV)-induced infectious mononucleosis (IM). They also demonstrated that cold agglutinins with equal reactivity against cord and adult RBCs were seen in 56 of 150 (37.3%) cases of heterophile-antibody-positive IM, in 1 of 7 (14.3%) cases of heterophile-antibody-negative EBV-induced IM and in 12 of 31 (38.7%) cases of heterophile-antibody-negative mononucleosis-like syndrome due to cytomegalovirus or other unspecified agents.

Anti-i is usually detected in the blood bank when a positive antibody screening is obtained, often due to an accompanying autoantibody of I or IH specificity. When a commercial reagent panel of group O adult RBCs is tested, varying degrees of reactivity are observed (primarily in the room temperature and/or immediate-spin phase) with weaker reactivity at 37 C. As mentioned before, expression of i antigen is enhanced in repeated phlebotomy, and this could explain why an example of anti-i could react strongly with a commercial reagent panel donor who is bled frequently. If cord RBCs are not used routinely in antibody identification, the presence or elucidation of anti-i specificity will go unrecognized. Most often the only clinical importance in identifying anti-i in a patient's serum would be as an aid to establishing a diagnosis of a disease associated with the presence of this antibody.

The i antigen is sometimes increased in Blackfan-Diamond syndrome, and the blood bank may receive a request for i typing on suspected cases. When testing a patient's RBCs for the i antigen, it is important to use anti-i of the same ABO group as the individual tested and control RBCs of the same ABO and approximate age. Not only is there variation in the i antigen on RBCs of the umbilical cord, the newborn, children and adults, but the antibody specificities may vary in sera (very few examples of anti-i are "pure"). It may very well be that some examples of anti-i used routinely are actually anti-Hi as described previously.[35(pp280-2),36(p79)]

In 1985, Shirey et al[39] reported an example of anti-i (in a patient with chronic PCH) that was a biphasic hemolysin. The direct antiglobulin test was positive with C3d coating the patient's RBCs. The patient's serum reacted only with i adult and cord RBCs. The reactions were strongest in indirect antiglobulin tests (IAT) at 4 C. The Donath-Landsteiner test was positive, and the anti-i acting as a biphasic hemolysin was detected only in the IgG fraction of the patient's serum.

In 1990, Judd et al[40] reported a case of anti-i that appeared to cause hemolysis after a negative immediate-spin crossmatch. The antibody screening was negative on pre- and posttransfusion sera, but transfusion reaction studies revealed that RBCs of one unit transfused reacted 1+ in LISS 37 C and 2+ in IgG IAT with both sera. Varying reactions were seen with reagent panel RBCs, but strong agglutination and hemolysis at 37 C was observed with cord and i adult RBCs. The investigators did point out that this anti-i is a unique cause of intravascular hemolysis of transfused RBCs and a rare cause of hemolysis due to anti-i when the antibody screening and immediate-spin crossmatch are negative.

Inhibition

HCF inhibits or partially inhibits some examples of anti-I and -i. Dzierzkowa-Borodej and coworkers[41] demonstrated presence of water-soluble I blood group substance in the saliva of all individuals, including newborn infants and i adults. Concentration of I substance varied from person to person.

Marsh et al[42] reported a higher concentration of I substance in human milk than in saliva. All anti-I sera were inhibited but to varying degrees not related to titer of the antibody. No difference was noted with I-inhibitory activity of milk due to variation in temperature (ie, inhibition at 4 C, 15 C, 23 C and 37 C). However, if the avidity of the antibody was first reduced by increasing the final reaction temperature, then inhibition by human milk was more effective. For instance, tests on inhibited serum showed only slight inhibition when tested at 4 C compared to a decrease in titer when tested at room temperature. Weak inhibition of anti-M, -P1 and -Lu^b was found, but if the pH of the treated milk was adjusted from pH 8.2 to 7.0 with phosphate buffer solution, the inhibitor effect on these antisera was abolished with no change in inhibitory effect on anti-I.

Appendix 5-3 outlines the procedure for inhibition of anti-I utilizing human breast milk.[30(pp115-6)] It should be pointed out that if anti-I and an uninhibitable antibody are present in the serum, reactivity in the test serum will be weaker than the control serum. Appropriate testing would then be done on the test serum to identify specificity of the "other" antibody.

Cooper[43] also investigated the inhibitory effect of human milk and other fluids, and found soluble I substance in human amniotic fluid and urine as well and confirmed its presence in milk. Inhibition of anti-I by amniotic fluid occurred very rapidly at 37 C and 4 C. Urine from adults, pregnant women and newborn babies contained inhibitory I substance but was of lesser potency than that found in amniotic fluid and milk. Saliva contained minimal inhibitory substance and cerebrospinal fluid had no activity.

Several studies have investigated the use of rabbit RBCs (which contain greater quantity of I antigen than human adult RBCs[44,45]) to adsorb cold autoagglutinins. Marks and coworkers[46] reported effective use of formaldehyde-fixed rabbit RBCs (FFRBC) to adsorb unwanted cold agglutinins. They found no reduction in reactivity of 19 alloantibodies from Rh, Kell, Duffy, Kidd and MNSs blood group systems when these were diluted 1 in 2 with three sera containing cold autoagglutinins.

Waligora and Edwards[47] carried their studies further by investigating the use of FFRBC and rabbit RBC stroma (RS) to adsorb cold autoagglutinins. They corroborated the findings of Marks et al but pointed out that several workers had previously found a B-like antigen on rabbit RBCs, and Waligora and Edwards could in most cases completely adsorb anti-B with FFRBC and RS. Thus, sera absorbed using this technique could not be used for serum grouping or compatibility testing. They also found some examples of anti-D, -E and -Le^{bH} that were either partially or completely absorbed. The procedure for absorption of cold autoantibody utilizing FFRBC or RS is outlined in Appendix 5-4.[30(pp82-3)]

In 1984, Weiland[48] examined 48 examples of anti-D and 25 examples of anti-E for a decrease in reaction strength following absorption with a commercial preparation of rabbit erythrocyte stroma. There was no significant decrease in titer endpoint or score of the antibodies following absorption.

However, in the reply by Edwards-Moulds and Waligora[49] to this letter, several important points were brought up. The commercial product was not used in their study so they could not comment on its performance. Their RS was prepared by digitonin lysis of washed rabbit RBCs. Adsorption with this RS reduced the titer of two of six saline examples of anti-D. They pointed out that variance in the data from Weiland's results and theirs could be due to the antibody class recognized by the techniques compared. Six of the eight examples of anti-D reacted at 24 C and presumably had an IgM component. Removal of IgM would not be obvious if only AHG titers were performed (as in Weiland's studies). They stated, "Although most clinically significant antibodies would be detected by AHG, we felt that 24 C tests were appropriate for two reasons: First the primary immune response often results in the production of IgM antibodies and, second, there are clinically significant antibodies reactive at 24 C (eg, anti-Tj^a, -Vel, -H)." In 1984 Ferrer and Cornwall[50] also responded to the recent publications with their observations that saline-agglutinating autoantibodies of Vel and PP$_1$P^k specificities were also absorbed by rabbit RBCs. They saw a 30-100% reduction in titration scores of saline-active anti-A, -B, -D, -E, -M, -N, -S, -P$_1$ and -PP$_1$P^k. They also cautioned users of FFRBC that more than anti-I can be removed from a serum.

One more report by Dzik et al[51] indicated that use of a commercial preparation of rabbit erythrocyte stroma interfered with the detection of anti-E and a warm-reactive anti-A$_1$, one or both of which resulted in a delayed transfusion reaction. A group A$_2$B previously transfused patient with a strong cold autoantibody (anti-HI), who initially had no alloantibodies (after successful cold autoabsorption), had a severe delayed hemolytic transfusion reaction 10 days after a series of transfusions. The posttransfusion DAT was positive, and both anti-A$_1$ and anti-E were present in the eluate. Serial serum samples had been treated with rabbit stroma and were used for antibody screening and compatibility testing before and during the reaction. Subsequent testing showed that both the anti-A$_1$ and -E were absorbed from the patient's serum with the rabbit stroma.

Inhibition and absorption techniques are useful in management of potent cold-reactive autoanti-I that interfere with screening for alloantibodies and subsequent compatibility testing. Both techniques have limitations—ie, not all sources of human milk are effective in inhibiting anti-I (one may work for one example and not another), and absorption with FFRBC or RS can remove some clinically significant alloantibodies from the patient's serum.

However, autoabsorption (the method of choice) cannot be done without risk of removing alloantibodies, if the patient has been recently transfused. Thus, inhibiting or absorbing the cold agglutinin may be better than doing nothing. Perhaps the technique of prewarming the serum would be effective in some instances when the cold agglutinin is not very strong. The procedure can be found in the 10th edition of the AABB *Technical Manual*.[17(pp555-6)] It should be pointed out it is recommended that the prewarmed test be incubated at 37 C for 30 minutes, since a potentiator is not added. An increased serum/cell ratio of 1:4 would also be useful in detecting weak alloantibodies.

Sd^a

Sd^a Antigen

The Sd^a antigen is absent on newborn (cord) RBCs and present on 91% of adult RBCs. The antigen on the RBCs is often lost in pregnancy. Cad+ RBCs, which are strongly agglutinated by *Dolichos biflorus* lectin, are extremely strong reactors with anti-Sd^a.[52] Association of Sd^a groups with ABO groups is apparent on RBCs, especially group A.[53]

In routine serologic testing, the antibody screening of a group A individual could be negative, but one of four crossmatches is weakly incompatible on immediate spin, 37 C and antiglobulin test. The most likely assumption is that the antibody is anti-A$_1$, but what happens if the patient is group A$_1$ and the autocontrol is nonreactive? Careful microscopic examination of reactivity with the group A incompatible unit will show the shiny orange-colored mixed-field refractile agglutination pattern typical of anti-Sd^a. If a commercial panel of group O RBCs is tested with the serum at room temperature for 30 minutes, spun and the tests read macroscopically and microscopically, the RBCs of a few donors should be agglutinated. If all are negative, then careful microscopic examination after incubation with the serum for 30 minutes at room temperature of the other three group A apparently "crossmatch-compatible" donors will surely demonstrate some reactivity with at least one or two of the donors.

Another example is a group O patient whose antibody screening is negative, and the RBCs of one of four donors are weakly reactive with the patient's serum. A commercial panel of 11 RBCs tested at room temperature for 30 minutes is also negative. Most likely the donor is strongly Sd(a+), and the antibody (anti-Sd^a) in the patient's serum is very weak. Testing the RBCs of the donor with *D. biflorus* lectin might show weak agglutination, indicating the donor is super Sd(a+) or even Cad+.

Sd^a is present in most human secretions in which ABH substance occurs, with only small amounts in saliva and large amounts in urine and meconium. Sd^a activity is present in the urine of several animal species with the guinea pig secreting 10 times as much Sd^a as any other species. Although the Sd^a RBC antigen is not present on cord RBCs and frequently lost in pregnancy, there appears to be little change in the amount of Sd^a in the urine.[54]

Anti-Sd^a

Anti-Sd^a is an IgM antibody that can be found in about 1% of the general population and may occur without previous stimulation by pregnancy or transfusion.[55,56] Some examples fix complement and can hemolyze enzyme pretreated RBCs. There is one report of an anti-Sd^a that caused a hemolytic transfusion reaction.[57] However, RBCs of the implicated donor gave a strong titer with the serum (512). The authors pointed out that reactions were seen with four of 58 cord samples. There is no mention in the report that it was ever shown that the patient was Sd(a−). The antibody could have been autoanti-Rx instead of anti-Sd^a.

The optimal phase of reactivity is saline RT (20 C), but some examples react only in the antiglobulin phase. The agglutination is classic and easily recognizable when reactions are observed microscopically; however, if screening and crossmatches are only read macroscopically some examples of anti-Sd^a go undetected.

Inhibition

In 1970, Morton and Terry[58] found Sd^a activity in urine of 96% of humans, and the same workers and Pickles reported that guinea pig kidney and urine were very rich in Sd^a.[59] In 1980 and 1981, Soh et al[60] and Morgan et al[61] demonstrated that Sd^a activity of urine is associated with human Tamm-Horsfall (T-H) glycoprotein, the most represented glycoprotein in urine. The procedure for inhibition of anti-Sd^a is outlined in Appendix 5-5.[30(pp120-1)] However, not included in the procedure is the instance when, if the test is weaker in reactivity than the control, the serum may contain inhibitable anti-Sd^a plus another uninhibitable antibody. A panel of reagent RBCs should be incubated with the test to identify the "other" antibody.

Also, in 1983 Judd[62] pointed out that before use, urine should be centrifuged or filtered and the pH adjusted to neutrality. The urine should then be dialyzed for 24-48 hours at 4 C against phosphate-buffered saline (pH 7.0-7.4). If this is not done, other antibodies could be nonspecifically inhibited [anti-Sd^x (Rx), -I, -i and LISS-dependent autoanti-P] due to variations in pH, osmolality and conductivity of urine.

In 1980, Marsh and coworkers[63] described two examples of an IgM saline-agglutining autoantibody they named anti-Sd^x because of similarities in reactivity to anti-Sd^a. The antibody was inhibited by human urine and strongly inhibited by guinea pig urine, but reacted with adult Sd(a−) and newborn RBCs. They reported that the antibodies appeared to be responsible for in vitro hemolysis of enzyme pretreated RBCs and in vivo hemolysis. The antibody activity was not cold-reactive, as incubation of the serum with test RBCs at 4 C did not increase the reactivity. In 1980 the authors encountered four additional examples of the antibody.

In 1983 Bass et al[64] investigated 12 examples of the antibody and showed that inhibition was due to a nonspecific effect caused by charged molecules. No specific urinary Sd^x substance could be demonstrated and they suggested that the antibody be renamed anti-Rx.

Serologically, the antibody reactivity was enhanced under acidic or low ionic conditions and suppressed in alkaline or high ionic conditions. Greatest serologic activity was seen by combining low pH and low ionic strength. All examples activated complement and gave in vitro and, in some cases, in vivo hemolysis. Anti-Rx has enhanced activity against neuraminidase-treated RBCs. The agglutinating activity is markedly affected by changes in salt concentration. One sample of guinea pig urine had acceptable pH and ionic values and had no anti-Sd^x substance. Their study showed consistent differences in conductivity of Sd(a+) and Sd(a−)

urine samples, but they pointed out that the Sd(a–) urine came from hospital patients. Since the urine inhibition of anti-Sd^x was due to a serologic artifact, there was no association to Sd^a and the antibody was renamed.

This author has investigated several examples of apparent autoanti-Rx, and although the name has been changed from Sd^x to Rx, there is still serologic similarity between the agglutination pattern of anti-Sd^a and -Rx. A few samples were referred to our Consultation Service specifically because microscopic examination revealed large shiny orange-colored agglutinates with a few free cells that resembled agglutination seen with anti-Sd^a. However, cord and Sd(a–) RBCs were reactive with the antibody, ruling out anti-Sd^a. It is important to differentiate between the two antibodies, since anti-Rx has been responsible for mild to severe hemolysis in vivo.

Pr

Antigens

Cold agglutinins (CA) not directed against Ii antigens react with Pr (protease-sensitive) antigens previously designated Sp$_1$ by Marsh[65] and HD by Roelcke[66] and consist of four related but different determinants—ie, Pr$_1$, Pr$_2$, Pr$_3$ and Pr^a. Primary serologic characteristics distinguishing Pr antigens from Ii are: 1) full expression on adult and newborn RBCs, 2) inactivation by proteases and 3) inactivation by neuraminidase (designated RDE for receptor destroying enzyme), except for Pr^a.[67]

Gd (glycolipid dependent), Sa, Fl, Lud and Vo are also N-acetylneuraminic acid (NeuAc)-dependent antigenic determinants on RBCs. Pr and Gd antigens are also on B and T lymphocytes and on phagocytic RBCs. Gd is also on platelets, and Gd and Sa antigens show different antigenic distribution patterns in human kidneys.[1(p295)]

Antibodies

The antibody specificities defining the Pr and Pr-related CA have been covered in the previous chapter. From a practical serologic standpoint it might be worthwhile to discuss how to recognize that a serum contains a Pr-related specificity and how to define the exact antigenic determinant recognized by the antibody.

In 1983, Roelcke and Kreft[67(pp210-3)] studied 41 examples of anti-Pr CA. Most (31 of 36) were IgM, although the first one described had been IgA. Subspecificities were defined by tests with untreated, protease-treated, neuraminidase (RDE)-treated human and animal RBCs. The subspecificities have been designated Pr$_{1h}$, Pr$_{1d}$, Pr$_2$, Pr$_{3h}$, Pr$_{3d}$ and Pr$_a$ (the h stands for human and d stands for dog; subspecificities of Pr_a are not well-defined and need further studies).

All were inhibited by a mixture of various sialoglycoproteins (SGPs) and some with purified glycophorin A (MN) SGP. En(a–) RBCs lacking glycophorin A react weakly but definitely with anti-Pr; thus, this is not the only SGP carrying Pr determinants. Pr antibodies can be distinguished from autoanti-En^a by lack of reactions with RDE-treated RBCs (except for anti-Pr_a). Anti-Pr_a is not as common as anti-Pr_1, -Pr_2 or -Pr_3, with only five found in the 35 sera tested. Twenty-five of the 35 were anti-Pr_1 and three were anti-Pr_2. Homozygous M^kM^k RBCs lacking glycophorin A and B do not react with Pr antibodies. It appears that both glycophorin A and B carry Pr determinants.

In 1985, McGinnis and coworkers described[68] a warm autoantibody most closely resembling anti-Pr_a, except for two exceptions. Most Pr_a antibodies are IgM, IgA or IgG CA, and their patient's antibody was a warm-reacting IgG antibody. Anti-Pr^a does not react with trypsin-treated RBCs, and their patient's antibody did.

Roelcke described[69] anti-Fl, a cold agglutinin recognizing a developmentally regulated antigen similar to I, but differing from I antigen since it was neuraminic acid (NeuAc) dependent. In 1984, Roelcke and Weber[70] encountered a patient's serum that contained both anti-Fl and anti-I CA. These specificities could be separated by absorption/elution procedures using neuraminidase (RDE)-treated RBCs. Reactions with the whole serum were indicative of anti-I, but after the serum was absorbed with RDE-treated RBCs, the serum contained reactivity for I adult RBCs, markedly weaker reactivity with newborn and i adult RBCs and no reactivity with RDE-treated RBCs (anti-Fl).

Roelcke showed that there appear to be different specificities of monoclonal anti-Gd CA.[71] Two showed preferential reactions with p RBCs and two did not. Anti-Fl and anti-Sa CA did not show preference for p RBCs.

Enzymes

Treatment of RBCs with proteases (ficin, papain, bromelin or trypsin) results in removal of sialic acid residues from the red cell membrane. Pr antigens are destroyed by protease treatment and Ii antigens are enhanced.

Appendices 5-6 and 5-7 outline procedures for treating RBCs with ficin, trypsin and papain.[29,72,73] Appendix 5-8 details the method for standardization of enzyme solutions.[74] Another good reference for use of enzymes in immunohematology is by Ellisor.[75]

Neuraminidase

Neuraminidase (RDE) cleaves sialic acid (NeuAc) from the red cell membrane but does not cleave protein. It reduces or destroys Pr antigens. Appendix 5-9 describes the procedure for treating RBCs with RDE.[72(p461)]

Inhibition

All anti-Pr CA are inhibited by human red cell SGPs. Increased inhibition is obtained after periodate oxidation and carbodiimide treatment of SGPs. None are inhibited by N-acetylneuraminic acid, and some are inhibited by sialyllactose.[67(p210)] RBC SGPs are prepared by the phenol/saline extraction method.[76] Peroxidase oxidation and carbodiimide treatment of SGPs are done by the methods of Suttajit and Winzler[77] and Roelcke et al.[78] McGinnis et al[68(p132)] summarize very well the methods for enzyme and neuraminidase treatment of RBCs, preparation of SGPs, inhibition techniques and serologic testing techniques.

Roelcke and Kreft[67(p210,212)] pointed out several important details to keep in mind when investigating CA.
1. It is sometimes difficult or even impossible to identify anti-Pr CA in whole sera. Anti-T must first be removed by absorption with RDE-treated RBCs.
2. Efficiency of RDE treatment must be demonstrated.
3. Contaminating anti-I may react with papain-treated and RDE-treated RBCs, partially or even completely masking the loss of anti-Pr reactivity.
4. Individual antibodies belonging to distinct specificities do not always express identical patterns. Thus, characterization of subspecificities should only be based on inhibition experiments with SGPs.

Summary

Cold agglutinins with P1, I and Sd^a specificity are commonly encountered in routine serologic testing in the blood bank. The P1 antigen varies from RBC to RBC, often making it difficult to elucidate this specificity, especially in combination with other alloantibodies. With the use of inhibition techniques, it becomes easier to resolve antibody problems involving anti-P1. Anti-I is usually an IgM autoantibody that can be absorbed from sera with rabbit RBCs and/or stroma, sometimes inhibited with human milk, and reactions can often be eliminated by use of a prewarming technique. Anti-Sd^a can be inhibited by human or guinea pig urine. Alloantibodies and autoantibodies of other specificities directed at antigens in the P and I blood groups are rare. But when they occur, it is good to have knowledge of various patterns of reactivity that give a clue to each specificity.

Anti-Rx and Pr-related antibodies are seen less frequently, and recognizing and resolving the specificities is less easily done than with P, I and Sd^a antibodies. Microscopic examination of tests with sera containing Rx antibodies reveals an agglutination pattern similar to Sd^a. Tests with enzyme-treated and RDE-treated RBCs can give a clue to presence of Pr antibodies. Studies confirming Pr specificities can then be done by testing animal, En(a−), M^{k}M^k RBCs, and inhibition with SGPs.

Although they are cold agglutinins, serologically these antibodies can interfere with routine compatibility testing and some may have the potential to be clinically significant. Hopefully, this chapter will provide a source for future reference in serologic management of these cold agglutinins.

References

1. Salmon C, Cartron JP, Rouger P. The human blood groups. New York: Mason Publishing USA Inc, 1984.
2. Tippett P. Contributions of monoclonal antibodies to understanding one new and some old blood group systems. In: Garratty G, ed. Red cell antigens and antibodies. Arlington, VA: American Association of Blood Banks 1986:86-93.
3. Cameron GL, Staveley JM. Blood group P substance in hydatid cyst fluids. Nature 1957;179:147-8.
4. François-Girard C, Gerday C, Beeley JG. Turtle-dove ovomucoid, a glycoprotein proteinase inhibitor with P$_1$ blood group activity. Biochem J 1979;177:679-85.
5. Radermecker M, Bruwier M, François C, et al. Anti-P activity in pigeon breeders' serum. Clin Exp Immunol 1975;22:546-9.
6. Ben-Ismail R, Rouger P, Carme B, et al. Comparative automated assay of anti-P$_1$ antibodies in acute hepatic distomiasis (fascioliasis) and in hydatidosis. Vox Sang 1980;38:165-8.
7. Bevan B, Hammond W, Clarke RL. Anti-P$_1$ associated with liver-fluke infection. Vox Sang 1970;18:188-9.
8. Norman P, MacIntyre D, Poole J, Mallan M. Allo-anti-P$_1$ in a P$_1$-positive person. Vox Sang 1985;49:211-14.
9. Tippett P, Sanger R, Race RR. An agglutinin associated with the P and ABO blood group systems. Vox Sang 1965;10:269-80.
10. Bruce M, Watt A, Gabra GS, et al. LKE red cell antigen and its relationship to P$_1$ and P^k: Serological study of a large family. Vox Sang 1988;55:237-40.
11. Vos GL, Celano MJ, Falkowski F, Levine P. Relationship of a hemolysin resembling anti-Tj^a to threatened abortion in Western Australia. Transfusion 1964;4:87-91.
12. Donath J, Landsteiner K. Über paroxysmale Hämoglobinurie. Münch med Wochenschr 1904;51:1590-3.

13. Weiner W, Gordon G, Rowe D. A Donath-Landsteiner antibody. Vox Sang 1964;9:684-97.
14. Worlledge S, Russo C. Studies on serology of paroxysmal cold haemoglobinuria (PCH), with special reference to its relationship with the P blood group system. Vox Sang 1965;10:293-8.
15. Ramos RR, Curtis BR, Eby CS, et al. Fatal autoimmune hemolytic anemia (AHA) associated with IgM bi-thermic anti-P and cold I^T (abstract). In: Book of abstracts from the ISBT/AABB Joint Congress. Arlington, VA: American Association of Blood Banks, 1990:86.
16. Dacie JV, Lewis SM. Practical hematology. 4th ed. London: Churchill, 1968.
17. Walker H, ed. Technical manual. 10th ed. Arlington, VA: American Association of Blood Banks, 1990:587-8.
18. Engelfriet CP, Beckers DO, von dem Borne AEGKr, et al. Haemolysins probably recognizing the antigen p. Vox Sang 1972;23:176-81.
19. Issitt CH, Duckett JB, Gut JB. A second example of anti-p (abstract). Transfusion 1975;15:521.
20. Allen FH Jr, Marsh WL, Jensen L, Finke J. Anti-IP: An antibody defining another product of interaction between the genes of the I and P blood group systems. Vox Sang 1974;27:442-6.
21. Issitt PD, Tegoli J, Jackson V, et al. Anti-IP_1: Antibodies that show an association between the I and P blood group systems. Vox Sang 1968;14:1-8.
22. Booth PB. Anti-I^TP_1: An antibody showing a further association between the I and P blood group systems. Vox Sang 1970;19:85-90.
23. McGinnis MH, Kaplan HS, Bowen AB, Schmidt PJ. Agglutinins for "null" red blood cells. Transfusion 1969;9:40-2.
24. Judd, WJ. A pH-dependent auto-agglutinin with anti-P specificity. Transfusion 1974;15:373-6.
25. Judd WJ, Steiner EA, Capps RD. Autoagglutinins with apparent anti-P specificity reactive only by low-ionic-strength salt techniques. Transfusion 1982;22:185-8.
26. Cohen DW, Nelson L. Auto-anti-P reacting only by low-ionic-strength solutions in a patient with hemolysis (letter). Transfusion 1983;23:79-80.
27. Tippett P, Wilfert K. Monoclonal anti-P_1 and anti-P^k antibodies (abstract). In: Proceedings of the Second International Workshop and Symposium on Monoclonal Antibodies Against Human Red Blood Cells and Related Antigens (Lund, Sweden). Paris: International Society of Blood Transfusion, 1990:91.
28. Cowles JW, Blumberg N. Neutralization of P blood group antibodies by synthetic solid-phase antigens. Transfusion 1987;27:272-5.
29. Skradski KJ. Application of inhibition technics. In: Rolih S, Albietz C, eds. Enzymes, inhibition and adsorptions. Washington, DC: American Association of Blood Banks, 1981:48-54.

30. Special techniques. Wallace ME, Green TS, eds. Selection of procedures for problem solving technical workshop. Arlington, VA: American Association of Blood Banks, 1983:77-145.
31. Marsh WL, Øyen R. A study of soluble Lewis and P_1 substances produced for use in immunohematology. Transfusion 1978;18:743-6.
32. Nelson WE, ed. Pediatrics. 12th ed. Philadelphia: WB Saunders Company, 1983.
33. Avery ME, Taeusch HW Jr. Diseases of the newborn. 5th ed. Philadelphia: WB Saunders Company, 1984.
34. Reviron M, Janvier D, Reviron J, Lagabrielle JF. An anti-I cold autoagglutinin enhanced in the presence of sodium azide. Vox Sang 1984;46:211-16.
35. Bird GWG, Wingham J. Erythrocyte autoantibody with unusual specificity. Vox Sang 1977;32:280-2.
36. Pierce SR, Kowalski MA, Hardman JT, Beck ML. Anti-Hi: More common than previously thought? (abstract). In: Book of abstracts from the ISBT/AABB Joint Congress. Arlington, VA: American Association of Blood Banks, 1990:79.
37. Dzierzkowa-Borodej W, Seyfried H, Lisowska E. Serological classification of anti-I sera. Vox Sang 1975;28:110-21.
38. Horowitz CA, Moulds J, Henle W, et al. Cold agglutinins in infectious mononucleosis and heterophil(sic)-antibody-negative mononucleosis-like syndromes. Blood 1977;50:195-202.
39. Shirey RS, Park K, Neso PM, et al. An anti-i biphasic hemolysin in chronic paroxysmal cold hemoglobinuria. Transfusion 1986;26:62-4.
40. Judd WJ, Steiner EA, Abruzzo L, et al. Anti-i causing acute hemolysis following a negative immediate-spin crossmatch (abstract). In: Book of abstracts from the ISBT/AABB Joint Congress. Arlington VA: American Association of Blood Banks, 1990:188.
41. Dzierzkowa-Borodej W, Seyfried H, Nichols M, Reid M. The recognition of water-soluble I blood group substance. Vox Sang 1970;18:222-34.
42. Marsh WL, Nichols ME, Allen FH Jr. Inhibition of anti-I sera by human milk. Vox Sang 1970;18:149-54.
43. Cooper AG. Soluble blood group I substance in human amniotic fluid. Nature 1970;227:508-9.
44. Moor-Jankowski J, Weiner AS, Gordon EB. Blood group antigens and cross reacting antibodies in primates, including man. Heterophile-like behavior of the blood group factor I. Exp Med Surg 1964;22:308-15.
45. Zelenski KS, Lambert RM. Blood group antigens I, i, H and HI on monkey, rabbit, and guinea pig erythrocytes. Proc Soc Exp Biol Med 1974;145:586-90.
46. Marks MR, Reid M, Ellisor SS. Absorption of unwanted cold autoagglutinins by formaldehyde-treated rabbit red blood cells (abstract). Transfusion 1980;20:629.

47. Waligora SK, Edwards JM. Use of rabbit red cells for adsorption of cold autoagglutinins. Transfusion 1983;23:328-30.
48. Weiland DL. Rabbit erythrocytes and stroma (letter). Transfusion 1984;24:369.
49. Edwards-Moulds J, Waligora SK. Rabbit erythrocytes and stroma (letter). Transfusion 1984;24:369.
50. Ferrer Z, Cornwall S. Absorption of saline agglutinins with rabbit red cells (letter). Transfusion 1984;24:541.
51. Dzik WH, Yang R, Blank J. Rabbit erythrocyte stroma treatment of serum interferes with recognition of delayed hemolytic transfusion reaction (letter). Transfusion 1986;26:303-4.
52. Sanger R, Gavin J, Tippett P, et al. Plant agglutinin for another human blood group. Lancet 1971;1:1130.
53. Giles CM. Antigens in plasma. In: Bell C, ed. A seminar on antigens on blood cells and body fluids. Washington, DC: American Association of Blood Banks, 1980:33-5.
54. Bird GW, Wingham J. The Cad/Sd^a blood groups. In: Seligson D, ed. CRC handbook series in clinical laboratory science. Vol. 1. Section D. Blood banking. Cleveland: CRC Press, Inc, 1977:455-70.
55. Macvie SI, Morton JA, Pickles MM. The reactions and inheritance of a new blood group antigen, Sd^a. Vox Sang 1967;13:485-92.
56. Renton PH, Howell P, Ikin EW, et al. Anti-Sd^a, a new blood group antibody. Vox Sang 1967;13:493-501.
57. Peetermans ME, Cole-Dergent J. Hemolytic transfusion reaction due to anti-Sd^a. Vox Sang 1970;18:67-70.
58. Morton JA, Terry AM. The Sd^a blood group antigen. Biochemical properties of urinary Sd^a. Vox Sang 1970;19:151-61.
59. Morton JA, Pickles MM, Terry AM. The Sd^a blood group antigen in tissues and body fluids. Vox Sang 1970;19:472-82.
60. Soh CPC, Morgan WTJ, Watkins WM, Donald ASR. The relationship between the N-acetylgalactosamine content and the blood group Sd^a activity of Tamm and Horsfall urinary glycoprotein. Biochem Biophys Res Commun 1980;93:1132-9.
61. Morgan WTJ, Soh CPC, Donald ASR, Watkins WM. Observations on the blood group Sd^a activity of Tamm-Horsfall urinary glycoprotein. Rev Fr Transf Immuno-hematol 1981;24:37-51.
62. Judd WJ. Urines for inhibition (letter). Transfusion 1983;23:404.
63. Marsh WL, Johnson CL, Øyen R, et al. Anti-Sd^x: A "new" auto-agglutinin related to the Sd^a blood group. Transfusion 1980;20:1-8.
64. Bass LS, Rao AH, Goldstein J, Marsh WL. The Sd^x antigen and antibody: Biochemical studies on the inhibitory property of human urine. Vox Sang 1983;44:191-6.
65. Marsh WL, Jenkins WJ. Anti-Sp$_1$: The recognition of a new cold auto-antibody. Vox Sang 1968;15:177-86.
66. Roelcke D. A new serological specificity in cold antibodies of high titre: Anti-HD. Vox Sang 1969;16:76-9.

67. Roelcke D, Kreft H. Characterization of various anti-Pr cold agglutinins. Vox Sang 1984;24:210-13.
68. McGinnis MH, Wasniowska K, Zopf DA, et al. An erythrocyte Pr auto-antibody with sialoglycoprotein specificity in a patient with purine nucleoside phosphorylase deficiency. Transfusion 1985;25: 131-6.
69. Roelcke D. A further cold agglutinin, Fl, recognizing a N-acetylneuraminic acid-determined antigen. Vox Sang 1981;41:98-101.
70. Roelcke D, Weber T. Simultaneous occurrence of anti-Fl and anti-I cold agglutinins in a patient's serum. Vox Sang 1984;47:122-4.
71. Roelcke D. Reaction of anti-Gd, anti-Fl and anti-Sa cold agglutinins with p erythrocytes. Vox Sang 1984;46:161-4.
72. Issitt PD. Applied blood group serology. 3rd ed. Miami: Montgomery Scientific Publications, 1985.
73. Low B. A practical method using papain and incomplete Rh-antibodies in routine Rh blood-grouping. Vox Sang 1955;5:94-8.
74. Widmann FK, ed. Technical manual. 9th ed. Arlington, VA: American Association of Blood Banks, 1985:425-6.
75. Ellisor SS. Action and application of enzymes in immunohematology. In: Bell CA, ed. A seminar on antigen-antibody reactions revisited. Arlington, VA: American Association of Blood Banks, 1982:133-74.
76. Baranowski T, Lisowska E, Morawiecki A, et al. Studies on blood group antigens M and N. III. Chemical composition of purified antigens. Arch Immunol Ther Exp 1959;7:15-27.
77. Suttajit M, Winzler RJ. Effect of modification of N-acetylneuraminic acid on the binding of glycoproteins to influenza virus and on susceptibility to cleavage by neuraminidase. J Biol Chem 1971;246: 3398-404.
78. Roelcke D, Ebert W, Geisen HP. Anti-Pr_3: Serological and immunochemical identification of a new anti-Pr subspecificity. Vox Sang 1976;30:122-33.

Appendix 5-1. Donath-Landsteiner Test[17]

Primary Application

The primary application of this test is in the differential diagnosis of immune hemolysis and paroxysmal cold hemoglobinuria (PCH). In particular, this procedure should be considered when cold-reactive autoantibodies are absent from the serum, C3 alone is present on the RBCs, the eluate is nonreactive and the patient has hemoglobinemia or hemoglobinuria, or both.

Materials

1. Serum to be tested, separated from a freshly collected blood sample maintained at 37 C.
2. Freshly collected normal serum as a source of complement.
3. 50% suspension of washed group O P+ RBCs (P_1 or P_2 phenotype).

Procedure

1. Label three sets of three 10 x 75-mm test tubes as follows: A1-A2-A3; B1-B2-B3; C1-C2-C3.
2. To tubes 1 and 2 of each set, add 10 volumes of patient's serum.
3. To tubes 2 and 3 of each set, add 10 volumes of fresh normal serum.
4. To all tubes, add one volume of washed 50% P+ RBCs and mix well.
5. Place the three "A" tubes first in a bath of melting ice for 30 minutes, and then at 37 C for 1 hour.
6. Place the three "B" tubes in a bath of melting ice, and keep them in melting ice for 90 minutes.
7. Place the three "C" tubes at 37 C, and keep them at 37 C for 90 minutes.
8. Centrifuge all tubes, and examine the supernatants for hemolysis.

Notes

1. To demonstrate the biphasic hemolysin associated with PCH, it is necessary to incubate the serum with RBCs first at or below 4 C, then at 37 C.
2. Complement is essential to demonstrate the antibody. Since patients with PCH often have low levels of serum complement, fresh normal serum should be included in the reaction medium as a source of complement.
3. To avoid loss of antibody by autoadsorption before testing, the patient's blood should be allowed to clot at 37 C, and the serum separated from the clot at 37 C.

Interpretation

The Donath-Landsteiner test, indicative of PCH, is considered positive when the patient's serum, with or without added complement, causes hemolysis only in those tubes that have been incubated first in melting ice and then at 37 C (ie, tubes A1 and/or A2). No hemolysis should be seen in any of the tubes maintained strictly at 37 C or in melting ice, or in which complement alone is present.

Reference

Dacie JV, Lewis SM. Practical hematology. 4th ed. London: Churchill; 1968.

Appendix 5-2. Inhibition of Anti-P1[30(pp 118-20)]

Purpose

To inhibit anti-P1, confirm the specificity and rule out or allow identification of other alloantibodies.

Principle

The P1 substance combines with the antibody in the test serum and agglutination due to anti-P1 cannot occur when P1+ RBCs are added to the treated serum.

Materials

1. Hydatid cyst fluid (HCF) (human or animal) containing scolices; or white of pigeon eggs.
2. pH 7.2 phosphate-buffered saline (PBS).
3. 0.85% NaCl (0.85 g/100 mL deionized water).

Procedure

Preparation of HCF

1. Fluid is extracted from the cyst and rendered noninfectious by incubating the fluid at 56 C for 1 hour.
2. One volume of HCF is mixed with nine volumes of PBS.
3. The buffered HCF can be stored in small aliquots at –20 C (or at 4 C if sterile filtered) until needed.

Preparation of Pigeon Egg White

1. Dilute with physiological saline until it is no longer viscous, yet still inhibits reactivity of anti-P1 (dilution of approximately 1 in 2000 or more).
2. If to be stored for future use, sterile filter and store in sterile vials at 4 C.

Test Procedure

1. Test—To one volume serum add one volume inhibiting fluid (HCF) or pigeon egg white.

2. Control—To one volume serum add one volume 0.85% NaCl.
3. Test and control sera are incubated at 20 C for 15-30 minutes.
4. Add appropriate RBC samples to test and control sera, and test at 20 C, 37 C and antiglobulin phases (if indicated).

Interpretation

1. Anti-P1 is present if no reactivity is observed in the test serum at 20 C and reactivity is seen in the control serum equivalent to the neat serum.
2. Anti-P1 is not present if reactivity in both test and control sera are equivalent to the neat serum.
3. Anti-P1 plus another antibody(ies) is indicated when reactivity in the test serum is weaker than reactivity in the control serum.
4. Dilution of the antibody has occurred rather than inhibition if no reactivity is observed in either the test or control sera.

Special Considerations

1. Test sera from #3 and #4 under Interpretation should be tested to identify underlying alloantibodies. Four drops of serum or a LISS technique can be used to increase sensitivity to compensate for dilution factor.
2. If anti-P1 is suspected based on strength of reactions with P1+ RBCs vs P1− RBCs, and strong reactions are observed in both test and control sera, the volume of P1 substance may not be adequate to inhibit the anti-P1. Two sets of serial dilutions of the serum in 0.85% NaCl should be set up—to one set add equal amount of inhibiting fluid and 0.85% NaCl to the other set.
3. Ratio of serum to P1 substance depends on strength of the antibody and amount of P1 substance in the inhibiting fluid.

Appendix 5-3. Inhibition of Anti-I[30(pp 115-16)]

Purpose

This procedure is utilized to inhibit anti-I reactivity in a test serum and allow identification of alloantibodies.

Principle

I substance, found in human milk, will combine with the corresponding antibody in the test serum, so that when I-positive red cells are added to the treated serum, agglutination due to anti-I cannot occur.

Materials

1. Human milk.
2. 0.85% NaCl (0.85 g/100 mL deionized water).
3. pH 7.2 phosphate-buffered saline (PBS).

Procedure

Preparation of Milk

1. Collect milk from lactating women into a clean container.
2. Centrifuge the milk for 10 minutes at 3600 rpm.
3. Remove and discard the cream layer.
4. Incubate the milk in boiling water for 10 minutes to inactivate the enzymes present.
5. Mix one volume of milk with one volume of pH 7.2 PBS. Freeze small aliquots and store at –20 C until needed.

Inhibition

1. Add one volume of the buffered milk to one volume of serum (Test).
2. Add one volume of 0.85% NaCl to another volume of serum (Control).
3. Incubate both the test and control sera at room temperature for 30 minutes.
4. Test the control and test sera with the appropriate red cell samples at the room temperature, 37 C and antiglobulin phases.

Interpretation

No reactivity in either the test or control sera—dilution of the antibody has occurred—no conclusion can be made.

Reactivity in both the test and control sera, equivalent to the neat serum—antibody is not anti-I.

No reactivity in the test serum and reactivity in the control serum equivalent to the neat serum—anti-I is present in the serum.

Notes

1. Anti-Le^a and anti-Le^b can also be inhibited if the milk is obtained from a Lewis-positive individual.
2. Twice as much (four drops instead of two) of the test and control sera can be added to each red cell sample to avoid dilution of the antibody specificities.
3. Strong reactions in both the test and control sera may indicate that the volume of I substance is not adequate to inhibit the antibody. Serial dilutions of the serum in 0.85% NaCl followed by the addition of an equal amount of buffered milk to one set of dilutions and an equal amount of 0.85% NaCl to another set of dilutions may be necessary to demonstrate inhibition.

References

1. Skradski KJ. Application of inhibition technics. In: Rolih S, Albietz C, eds. Enzymes, inhibitions and adsorptions. Washington, DC: American Association of Blood Banks, 1981:51-2.
2. McKeever BG. Antibody screening and identification. In: Treacy M, Smith MJ, eds. Pretransfusion testing for the '80s. Washington, DC: American Association of Blood Banks, 1980:64-7.

Appendix 5-4. Cold Autoantibody Absorption With Formaldehyde-Fixed Rabbit Red Blood Cells or Rabbit Stroma[30(pp 82-83)]

Purpose

This procedure is used to remove cold autoagglutinins from sera. It is particularly useful when autoabsorption cannot be safely performed in a recently transfused individual. It is also useful when the patient has a very low hematocrit and there is not a sufficient quantity of patient red cells to remove a strong cold autoagglutinin. Removal of the cold autoantibody allows for better and easier identification of accompanying alloantibodies.

Principle

Rabbit red cells have a greater amount of I antigen than human adult red cells. The rabbit cells are fixed with formaldehyde to preserve the cells for future absorption studies.

Materials

1. Formaldehyde-fixed rabbit cells (FFRBC)
   a. Clotted rabbit cells are pooled, homogenized in blender, filtered through gauze and washed with 0.9% saline.
   b. Working formaldehyde solution consists of one part of stock 40% solution to 39 parts of 0.9% saline. The pH is adjusted to 7.2 using 1 N NaOH.
   c. Rabbit red cells are fixed by adding two parts of the working formaldehyde to one part of washed red cells and incubating at 37 C for 72 hours.
   d. The fixed red cells are washed six times in 0.9% saline and stored at 24 C.
2. If rabbit stroma (RS) is desired, lyse the washed rabbit red cells with digitonin.

Procedure

1. One mL of serum is mixed with two mL FFRBC or 0.5 mL of stroma.
2. Incubate mixtures at 4 C ± 2 for 60 minutes and remove absorbed serum after centrifugation.
3. Test absorbed serum at room temperature, 37 C and AHGT (not 4 C) against appropriate test red cells.

Interpretation

1. If no agglutination is detected in the absorbed serum, the procedure effectively removed the cold autoagglutinin.
2. If there is still agglutination in any of the routine phases of testing, the cold autoagglutinin may not have been completely removed from the serum or there is an accompanying alloantibody.

Comments

1. Both FFRBC and RS are equally effective in removing all antibody activity in 92% of cases studied.
2. However, some alloantibodies such as anti-D, anti-E and anti-Le^b are also reduced in titer or completely removed.[1]
3. Anti-B will be completely absorbed by FFRBC and RS in most cases.[2] Thus, sera absorbed with rabbit red cells or stroma would be contraindicated for serum ABO grouping. This should be kept in mind in compatibility testing.

References

1. Marks MR, Reid M, Ellisor SS. Adsorption of unwanted cold autoagglutinins by formaldehyde treated rabbit red blood cells (abstract). Transfusion 1980; 20:629.
2. Waligora SK, Edwards JM. The use of rabbit red blood cells for the adsorption of cold autoagglutinins. Transfusion 1983;23:328-30.

Appendix 5-5. Inhibition of Anti-Sd^a [30(pp 120-1)]

Purpose

This procedure is utilized to inhibit the reactivity in a test serum due to a suspected anti-Sd^a and to allow identification of any other alloantibodies.

Principle

Sd^a substance, found in the urine of an Sd(a+) individual or in a guinea pig urine, will combine with the corresponding antibody in a test serum, so that when Sd(a+) red cells are added to the treated serum, agglutination due to the anti-Sd^a cannot occur.

Materials

1. Urine from an Sd(a+) individual.
2. Urine from an Sd(a−) individual.
3. 0.85% NaCl (0.85 g/100 mL deionized water).
4. pH 7.4 phosphate-buffered saline (PBS).

Procedure

Preparation of Urine Specimens

1. Select donors who are Sd(a+) to obtain urine rich in Sd^a substances. Select a donor who has produced anti-Sd^a to obtain urine lacking Sd^a substance.
2. Obtain a cleanly voided urine specimen.
3. Centrifuge urine specimen.
4. Dilute each urine specimen with an equal amount of pH 7.4 PBS. (Urine specimens may be extremely acidic and this dilution is necessary to prevent hemolysis of test red cells.)
5. Aliquots of diluted urines can be frozen until needed.

Inhibition

1. Add one volume of diluted Sd(a+) urine to one volume of serum (Test).
2. Add one volume of diluted Sd(a−) urine to another volume of serum (Control). [If Sd(a−) urine is not available, 0.85% NaCl may be used instead.]
3. Incubate both test and control sera at room temperature for 30 minutes.

4. Test the control and test sera with appropriate red cell samples at the room temperature, 37 C and antiglobulin phases.

Interpretation

1. No reactivity in either the test or control sera indicates a dilution of the antibody has occurred and no conclusion can be made.
2. Reactivity in both the test and control sera equivalent to the neat serum indicates that the antibody is not anti-Sd^a.
3. No reactivity in the test serum and reactivity in the control serum equivalent to the neat serum indicate the presence of anti-Sd^a in the serum.

Notes

1. Twice as much (four drops instead of two) of the test and control sera can be added to each red cell sample to avoid dilution of antibody specificities.
2. Strong reactions in both the test and control serum may indicate that the volume of Sd^a substance is not adequate to inhibit the antibody. Serial dilutions of the serum in 0.85% NaCl followed by the addition of an equal amount of Sd(a+) urine to one set of dilutions and an equal amount of Sd(a–) urine to another set of dilutions may be necessary to demonstrate inhibition.

Reference

McKeever BG. Antibody screening and identification. In: Treacy M, Smith MJ, eds. Pretransfusion testing for the '80s. Washington, DC: American Association of Blood Banks, 1980:63-7.

Appendix 5-6. Preparation of Ficin and Trypsin[29(pp 20-2),72]

Preparation of Ficin

Preparation of Stock 1% Ficin Solution

1. Mix 1.0 gram of ficin in 100 mL of pH 7.3 buffered saline.
2. Agitate the mixture for 15 minutes at room temperature.
3. Centrifuge the solution at 1000 g for 5 minutes.
4. Transfer supernatant to a small tube (1 mL aliquots) and store at –20 C or below.
   Note: Some people may have dangerous hypersensitivity to ficin powder; they should work with the powder under a hood and wear gloves.

Preparation of Working 0.1% Ficin Solution

Mix 1 volume of the 1% ficin stock solution with 9 volumes of pH 7.3 buffered saline. Prepare fresh each day of use.

Preparation of Trypsin

Reagents

1. 0.1 M phosphate buffer pH 7.7.
   Mix 9 mL of 0.1 M Na_2HPO_4 and 1.0 mL of 0.1 M KH_2PO_4. Check pH and adjust if necessary.
2. 10 mL of 0.05 M HCl.
3. Crystalline trypsin Type III 2X crystallized or crude trypsin powder.

Procedure

1. Dissolve 0.1 gram of crystalline trypsin in 10 mL of 0.05 M HCl, OR dissolve 2.5 grams of trypsin powder in 10 mL of 0.05 M HCl.
2. Mix and incubate at 4 C for 24 hours. Mix periodically.
3. Centrifuge or filter and dispense into small aliquots. Store at –20 C.
   Note: Trypsin powder may also contain chymotrypsin.

Appendix 5-7. Preparation of Löw's Cysteine-Activated Papain[29(p 21),73]

Reagents

1. 0.067 M phosphate buffer pH 5.4
   Mix 15 mL of 0.007 M Na_2HPO_4 (9.46 g/L) and 5000 mL of 0.067 M KH_3PO_4 (9.07 g/L). Check and adjust pH if necessary.
2. 0.5 M L-Cysteine hydrochloride hydrate
   Dissolve 1.2 g of L-cysteine HCL in 20 mL of distilled H_2O.
3. Papain, crude powder.

Preparation of Stock Papain Solution

1. Grind 1 gram of papain with a small volume of the 0.067 M phosphate buffer pH 5.4 in a mortar.
2. Transfer suspension quantitatively to 500 mL graduated mixing cylinder using the buffer as a wash.
3. Make up to 380 mL with buffer.
4. Add 0.5 M L-cysteine solution (20 mL).
5. Transfer to a 500 mL flask, cover and incubate in a 37 C waterbath for 1 hour.
6. Centrifuge or filter and dispense into small aliquots. Store at –20 C.

Note

1. This is Löw's original procedure and results in a 0.25% papain solution.
2. Papain is not stable at 4 C. Papain should be thawed just prior to use and stored at 4 C for no longer than 12 hours.
3. Cysteine-activated papain may cause slight discoloration of reagent red cells.

Appendix 5-8. Standardization of Enzyme Solutions for Two-Stage Technique[74]

Principle

The amount of enzymatic activity varies each time a batch of stock enzyme solution is prepared. To eliminate this variable in serological testing each new batch of enzyme stock solution should be tested with known antibodies (a dilute Rh antibody and a potent anti-Fy^a). The incubation time or if necessary the concentration of the working solution should be varied until results similar to the previous working enzyme solution are obtained.

Reagents

1. New batch of stock enzyme.
2. Sera from patients with negative antibody screens.
3. Weak anti-D that will agglutinate enzyme treated D+ cells but not untreated cells at 37 C.
4. A potent (2–3+) anti-Fy^a.

Procedure

1. Dilute stock enzyme solution to the appropriate working dilution.
2. Label three tubes: 5 minutes, 10 minutes and 15 minutes.
3. Add equal volume of washed packed red cells and working enzyme solution to each tube.
4. Incubate for the designated time at 37 C. Wash the cells 3 times and resuspend the cells to a 2-3% cell suspension.
5. For each serum to be tested (negative controls, anti-D and anti-Fy^a) label four tubes: untreated, 5 minutes, 10 minutes and 15 minutes.
6. Add 1 drop of the appropriate cell suspension to each tube.
7. Add 2 drops of the serum to be tested.
8. Mix and incubate for 15 minutes at 37 C.
9. Centrifuge and read for agglutination.
10. Wash cells 4 times and perform indirect antiglobulin test.

Interpretation

1. The optimum incubation time is the one that exhibits the greatest reactivity with the dilute anti-D; no reactivity with the anti-Fy^a; and finally no nonspecific agglutination with the negative sera.

2. If necessary, adjust the concentration of the working solution to achieve the desired results.

Notes

1. Avoid changing the concentration of the working enzyme solution, if possible. Any stock solution that requires a drastic change from the previous enzyme solution should be discarded and a new batch of stock solution made and tested.
2. If routine technique uses 1 drop of 2-3% cell suspension instead of equal volume of packed cells, the above procedure should be modified accordingly, so that the enzyme is evaluated by the technique routinely used.

Appendix 5-9. Neuraminidase Treatment of Red Cells[72]

Principle

Neuraminidase is an exoglycosidase that specifically cleaves sialic acid (NeuAc) from the red cell membrane. Unlike ficin, trypsin and papain (which are proteases), neuraminidase does not cleave protein so the effect of this enzyme on the red cell is limited and very specific. Exposure of a red cell to neuraminidase will expose cryptic antigens such as T and reduce or destroy the M, N and Sp-Pr antigens.

Reagents

1. Neuraminidase B grade (can be obtained from Calbiochem or Grand Island Biologicals). Note the activity given is international units (IU).
2. Phosphate-buffered saline pH 7.3.

Procedure A: 40% Reduction in Sialic Acid (NeuAc)

1. Wash cells 3 times and prepare 12 mL of a 25% cell suspension.
2. Dilute small aliquot of neuraminidase with PBS to give 1 IU/mL.
3. Add 20 lambda of the diluted neuraminidase.
4. Mix and incubate at 37 C for 30 minutes.
5. Wash cells 3 times with isotonic saline and resuspend to a 3-4% cell suspension.
6. Test cells with *Arachis hypogea* lectin to determine if the cells have been T-activated.

Procedure B: 80% Reduction in Sialic Acid (NeuAc)

1. Resuspend 1 mL of washed packed cells to a 20% cell suspension with PBS pH 7.3.
2. Prepare neuraminidase as in Step 2 above.
3. Add 0.2 mL of diluted neuraminidase.
4. Incubate at 37 C for 30 minutes.
5. Continue as in Procedure A.

Notes

1. Some investigators recommend adding $CaCl_2$ (to final concentration of 0.001 M) to the cell-enzyme mixture for optimal T-activation.
2. All normal adult sera contains naturally occurring anti-T.

Index

(Italicized page numbers indicate tables or figures.)

A
ABH
 I, and P complexes, 29-32
 Ii, 33
Abortion, spontaneous, anti-$P+P_1+P^k$, 17
Agglutinin disease, cold, anti-I, *37*
Agglutinins, cold, 23
 non-Pr antigens, 88-95
 other disease associations, 41-42
 unnamed antigens defined by, 101
Aging, Ii antigens, 24-25
Anemia
 hemolytic, anti-Pr, 78-79
 Ii antigens, 42
Antibodies
 drug-induced, hemolysis and, 44
 polyclonal, 15
 See also particular antibody
Antibodies, monoclonal
 anti-Pr, 87-88
 P, 116
Antigens
 unnamed, defined by cold agglutinins, 101
 See also particular antigen
Autoagglutinins, cold, infections, 40
Autoantibodies
 absorption, cold, 139-140
 cold-reactive, I and P blood groups, 72-112
 I, 121
 P, 115-116
 Pr, 78
 Sd^a, 124

B
Blackfan-Diamond syndrome, i antigen, 119-120
Blacks, P system phenotypes, 10, *11*

C
Cad antigen, 53, 60-*61*
 biochemistry, *61*, 64-65
 Dolichos biflorus, 60
 Sd^a same as?, 65-67
 structure, 64-65
Cataracts, Ii antigens, 43-44
CDH. *See* Ceramide dihexoside
Ceramide dihexoside, 3, 6-*8*-*9*-10

Ceramide precursors, 5
Ceramide trihexoside, 3, 6-*8*-*9*-10
CHD. *See* Hemagglutinin disease, cold
Coxsackie A, cold autoagglutinins, 40
CTH. *See* Ceramide trihexoside

D
Disease
 Ii antigens, 42-44
 See also Immunology; Infection
Dolichos biflorus
 anti-Sd^a, 62
 Cad antigen, 60
Donath-Landsteiner antibody
 PCH, 17-18, 115
 test, 133-134
Drug-antibody complexes, Ii antigens, 44

E
En^a antibody, differentiation between anti-Pr, 84-85
Enzyme solutions, two-stage technique, standardization, 145-146
Epstein-Barr virus, anti-I, 39-40
Erythropoiesis, Ii antigens, 43

F
Ficin preparation, 143
Fl antigen, 91-92, 95, *96, 98, 99*
Forssman antigen, 3, *5*

G
Gd antigen, 89-90, 95, *96, 98, 99*
 CHD, 89
Genetics
 Ii blood groups, 32-34
 P blood group, 6-*8*-*9*-*11*-15
Genotypes, P system, *11*
Globoside series, 3, *5*
Glycosphingolipids, 3, *4*
Glycosyltransferases, 7

H
HCF, anti-I, 120
H chains, Ii activity, *33*
Hemagglutination, Ii antigens and temperature, 34-35
Hemagglutinin disease, cold
 anti-Pr, 85-86
 Gd antigen, 89
 I and P blood groups, 72, 79
 Ii blood groups, 35-36

149

MoAbs, 87-88
Sa antigen, 90
Hemoglobinuria, paroxysmal cold
  auto-anti-P, 17-18
  Donath-Landsteiner antibody, 115
  I and P blood groups, 72, 79
Hemolysis, drug-induced antibodies, and, 44
H(i), 30-31
Hi antibody, typical reactions, *31*

I

ABH, and P complexes, 29-32
serologic history, 24-*25*-29
serology, 117-122
I antibody, 118-120
  cold agglutinin disease, *37*
  EBV, 39-40
  infections, other, 40
  inhibitable and noninhibitable, 28
  inhibition, 120-122, 137-138
  Mycoplasma pneumoniae infection, 38-39
  typical benign and pathogenic examples, 36-*37*-38
  typical reactions at 4 C, *25*
I antigens, 117
  autoantibody, 118, 119, 121
I blood group, 23-52
  cold-reactive autoantibodies, 72-112
i antibody, 119-120
  disease associations, 41-42
i serologic history, 24-*25*-29
IA, 29
IA antibody, typical reactions at 4 C, *29*
IB, 29-30
IB antibody, typical reactions at 4 C, *30*
I^D, 28
I^F, 28
IgM^{woo} antibody, 93, 95, *97-99*
IH, 30-31
iH, 31
Ii antibodies, infections, 38-42
Ii antigens
  aging, 24-25
  disease associations, 42-44
  drug-antibody complexes, 44
  hemagglutination and temperature, 34-35
Ii blood groups
  biochemistry, 32-34
  genetics, 32-34
  H chains, <u>34</u>
  pathologic significance, 35-44
  serologic heterogeneity 26
  subspecificities, 26-29
ILe^{bH}, 32

Immunology
  anti-Pr, 85-88
  See also Disease; Infection
In(Lu) and P1 antigen, 12
Infections
  autogglutinins, cold, 40
  Ii antibodies, 38-42
  See also Disease; Immunology
IP_1, 32
I^S, 28-29
I^T, 26-28
I^T antibody, 119
  disease associations, 41
  typical reactions at 4 C *27*

J-L

Ju antigen, 94-95, *97, 99*
Leukemia, Ii antigens, 43
Li antigen, 93, 95, *97, 98, 99*
Listeria monocytogenes, anti-I, 41
LKE. *See* Luke
Lud antigen, 92, 95, *96, 98, 99*
Luke antibody, 11-12, 114-115
Luke antigen, 11-12, 113

M

Malignant disease, $P+P_1+P^k$ antibody, 16
Me antigen, 93-9495, *97, 99*
Milk, human, anti-I, 120-121
Mycoplasma pneumoniae infection, anti-I, 38-39

N-O

Neuraminidase, Pr, 127
  treatment of red cells, 147
O(i), 30-31
Om antigen, 94, 95, *97, 99*

P

ABH, and I complexes, 29-32
  MoAbs, 116
  serology, 113-117
P antibody, 14
  human, 114-116
  inhibition, 117
P antigens, 113-114
P autoantibody, PCH, 17-18
P blood group system, 1-22
  biochemistry, 2-3
  clinical significance, 15-19
  cold-reactive autoantibodies, 72-112
  genetics, 6-*8-9-11*-15
  phenotypes, 10, *11*
  urinary tract infection, 18-19
p antibody, 15
p determinant, *6*
$P+P_1+P^k$, abortion, spontaneous, 17

P+P$_1$+P^k antibody, 14-15
   malignant disease, 16
P1, 1
P1 antibody, 12-*13*-14
   inhibition, 135-136
   transfusion practice, 15-16
P1 antigen
   distribution, 2
   In(Lu), 12
   red cells, *9*
   structure, 3-*4-5-6*
Papain, Low's cysteine-activated, preparation, 144
Paragloboside series, 3, *6*
PCH. *See* Hemoglobinuria, paroxysmal cold
Phenotypes, P system, *11*
Pr
   determinants, possible sites, 83-84
   enzymes, 126
   serology, 125-127
Pr antibodies, 125-126
   anti-En^a, differentiation between, 84-85
   hemolytic anemia, 78-79
   idiotypes, 86-87
   immunology, 85-88
   inhibition and enhancement, *82*, 127
   MoAbs, 87-88
   red cell clearance, 88
   serology, 74-79
   subspecificities, typical reactions, *76-77*
Pr antigens, 73-88, 95-*96, 98, 99*, 125
   biochemistry, 79-84
   serology, 74-79
Pr autoantibodies, 78
Pr$_1$ antigen, 75
   biochemistry, 79-81
Pr$_2$ antigen, 75
   biochemistry, 79-81
Pr$_3$ antigen, 75
   biochemistry, 79-81
Pr$_a$, 82
Pr$_a$ antigen, 75
Pregnancy, Sd^a, 56

Pr^M, 82-83
Pr^M antigen, 75
Pr^N, 82-83
Pr^N antigen, 75

R

Red blood cells, Sd^a antigens, 54-55
Red cell clearance, anti-Pr, 88
Rx antigen, 98, 100

S

Sa antigen, 90-91, 95, *96, 98, 99*
   CHD, 90
Sd^a
   biochemistry 61-*63*
   Cad same as?, 65-67
   other findings, 59
   phenotypes, *55*
   serology, 122-125
   sources of soluble, 55-56
Sd^a antibody, 123-124
   clinical significance, 58-59
   detection, 56-57
   inhibition, 124-125, 141-142
   structure, 62-*63*
Sd^a antigen, 52-59, 122-123
   RBCs, 54-55
Sialosylparagloboside, *6*
Sickle cell anemia, Ii antigens, 43

T-W

Temperature, Ii antigens and hemagglutination, 34-35
Tetrasaccharides, *80-81*
Tj^a antibody, 14-15
Transfusion practice, P1 antibody, 15-16
Trisaccharides, *80-81*
Trypsin preparation, 143
Urinary tract infection, P blood group, 18-19
Vo antigen, 93, 95, *96, 98, 99*
Whites, P system phenotypes, 10, *11*